Clinical Management of Prostatic Cancer

Titles of Related Interest

Soloway, Hardeman/*Clinical Management of
Bladder Cancer*
Publication 1989

Other titles under development:

Clinical Management of Testicular Cancer
Clinical Management of Renal (Cell) Cancer

Clinical Management of Prostatic Cancer

JOSEPH A. SMITH, JR., M.D.
Associate Professor
Division of Urology
Department of Surgery
University of Utah School of Medicine
Salt Lake City, Utah

RICHARD G. MIDDLETON, M.D.
Chairman, Division of Urology
University of Utah School of Medicine
Salt Lake City, Utah

YEAR BOOK MEDICAL PUBLISHERS, INC.
Chicago • London • Boca Raton

1 2 3 4 5 6 7 8 9 0 KC 91 90 89 88 87

Library of Congress Cataloging-in-Publication Data

Smith, Joseph A., 1949–
   Clinical management of prostatic cancer.

   Includes bibliographies and index.
   1. Prostate gland—Cancer.   I. Middleton, Richard G.
II. Title.   [DNLM: 1. Prostatic Neoplasms—therapy.
WJ 752 S651c]
RC280.P7S65   1987   616.99'463   87-6129
ISBN 0-8151-7843-3

Sponsoring Editor: Daniel J. Doody
Manager, Copyediting Services: Frances M. Perveiler
Production Project Manager: Carol A. Reynolds
Proofroom Supervisor: Shirley E. Taylor

Preface

The subject of prostatic cancer has been addressed extensively in the medical literature. To a great extent, interest has been prompted by the frequency of the disease as well as the intriguing and unpredictable natural history of prostatic cancer in an individual patient. In addition, the large body of printed literature as well as verbal discussion generated by carcinoma of the prostate have emerged because of the strikingly different—and often opposing—viewpoints regarding appropriate treatment in a given clinical situation. Because of this, the clinician frequently is both frustrated and confused in attempting to make clinical decisions or treatment recommendations for patients with prostatic cancer.

It is not the purpose of this book to review exhaustively the literature on prostatic cancer or simply to reproduce information that is otherwise easily obtainable. Rather, an attempt is made to present practical, reasonable recommendations based on extensive clinical experience as well as interpretation of the pertinent literature. Thus, this book is intended for all clinicians involved in the treatment of patients with prostatic cancer.

Considering the confusing and sometimes contradictory data that have been generated regarding prostatic cancer, dogmatic treatment recommendations frequently are unfounded and often reflect a poor understanding of the disease. Therefore, alternative treatment approaches are acknowledged as much as possible. To a great extent, therapeutic recommendations should be based on efforts to select patients most likely to benefit from a given form of treatment, while sparing treatment expense and morbidity in those patients unlikely to respond or not in need of treatment.

Inevitably, some of our biases emerge through some of the treatment recommendations. Clinical biases cannot be completely subdued but should be based as much as possible upon an impartial and objective interpretation of available information as well as application of these data to the circumstances of an individual situation. A simple presentation of facts and "letting the patient make the choice" is impractical and often unfair to patients. Although patient wishes are paramount in deciding upon treatment, the very basis of clinical skill is to weigh the advantages and disadvantages of a given treatment and present the options and recommendations to a patient in a meaningful manner. In this way, the most appropriate treatment in terms of both therapeutic efficacy and treatment morbidity can be determined for an individual patient.

Sincere appreciation is expressed to Marcia Thompson for her usual excellent work in the preparation of this text.

JOSEPH A. SMITH, JR., M.D.
RICHARD G. MIDDLETON, M.D.

Contents

1

Detection and Diagnosis

EPIDEMIOLOGY

In the United States and many European countries, carcinoma of the prostate is the second most common cancer and the third leading cause of cancer death in men. In the United States alone, it is estimated by the American Cancer Society that there will be 90,000 new cases of prostatic cancer in 1986 and 26,000 deaths.[1] Although the etiology of prostatic cancer is unknown, some contributing factors to the development of the disease have been defined as well as some dominant epidemiologic patterns. A general knowledge of these factors is important for the clinician treating patients with prostatic cancer because it may help identify individual patients or segments of the population at large who may be at greater risk and require more careful screening or follow-up.

Age

The association between prostatic cancer and increasing age is well recognized and striking. Unlike most cancers which may have a peak age of incidence, the incidence and prevalence of prostatic cancer continue to increase with advancing age. Autopsy studies have shown histologic evidence of prostatic cancer in over 40% of men whose death occurs in the ninth decade.[2]

Equally impressive is the low incidence of the disease below age 50 or 55. Prostatic cancer is a rare disease in younger men. In general, it is recommended that yearly rectal examination for screening of prostatic cancer begin at age 50 in most men. A widespread clinical impression among physicians treating prostatic cancer is that the disease is more virulent and rapidly progressive in younger men. Although statistical studies do not necessarily verify this impression on a stage-for-stage basis, they do indicate that metastatic disease is found more often at the time of presentation in younger men than in older age groups.[3] Finally, it is anticipated that the disease will have a clinically significant impact or eventually be the cause of death for a greater percentage of younger men in whom longevity would otherwise be greater.

1

Race

In epidemiologic studies of cancer, it is difficult to separate racial factors from other influences. Culture, diet, and environment vary among ethnic or racial groups even within the same country. Nevertheless, there are striking differences in the incidence of prostatic cancer that are notable on a worldwide basis and among ethnic groups within the same country. Curiously, most studies suggest that the prevalence of clinically occult prostatic cancer found at autopsy is similar throughout all countries and racial groups.[4] However, the rates of clinically apparent disease and prostatic cancer mortality vary widely.

The highest incidence of age-adjusted death rate from prostatic cancer is found in Scandinavian countries (Fig 1–1). The United States has an incidence similar to that of most Northern European countries, whereas rates are somewhat lower in Israel, southern Europe, and South America. The lowest reported incidence of prostatic cancer occurs in Oriental countries. Some of these differences may be artifactual and related to variability in reporting of prostatic cancer. Decreased overall life expectancy in some countries may also be contributory. Within the United States, prostatic cancer occurs most commonly in blacks.[5] Overall mortality is increased in blacks compared to white populations, and metastatic disease is evident more often at the time of presentation.

Some of the more interesting studies regarding the influence of race and

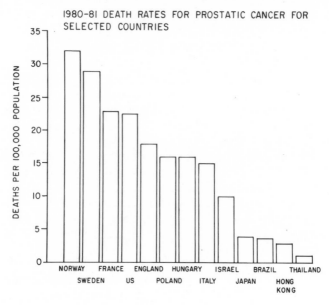

FIG 1–1.
Graph showing relative incidence of prostatic cancer for selected countries. Overall, clinically apparent prostatic cancer is most common in Scandinavian countries and least common in Oriental countries.

environment on prostatic cancer have involved populations of Japanese patients. Although the incidence of clinically apparent carcinoma of the prostate is relatively low in Japan and in first-generation Japanese migrants to the continental United States, the mortality from prostatic cancer rises in Japanese Americans living in the continental United States for more than one generation.[6] Similarly, the proliferative type of latent prostatic cancer is seen with increased frequency in Japanese migrants to Hawaii compared to those in Japan.[7] Thus, although race alone seems to be a factor influencing the frequency of prostatic cancer, these studies underscore the obvious additional impact of environmental factors.

Familial Factors

Carcinoma of the prostate occurs more frequently in the sons and siblings of patients who have developed clinically apparent disease (Table 1–1). A fourfold increase in the incidence of prostatic cancer occurs in the brothers of patients who develop the disease by the seventh decade of life.[8] Whether this indicates a genetic predisposition for prostatic cancer or is simply a reflection of exposure to similar environmental influences is uncertain. However, sons of patients with prostatic cancer have been found to have circulating serum testosterone levels that are somewhat lower than those of a control population with no family history of prostatic cancer.[8] The interpretation and significance of these studies is difficult to determine, but they do underscore the wisdom of a screening rectal examination and careful follow-up of male family members of patients with prostatic cancer.

Previous Prostatic Disease

A common concern among men with nonmalignant diseases of the prostate or genitourinary tract is the possible association between these problems and the subsequent development of carcinoma. The frequency of occurrence

TABLE 1–1.
Risk of Prostatic Cancer for Brothers of Patients With Known Prostatic Cancer*†

	AGE, YEAR						
	50–54	55–59	60–64	65–69	70–74	75–79	80–84
Cumulative risk of developing prostatic cancer							
Brothers	0.004	0.020	0.033	0.081	0.204	0.528	0.528
Control population (State of Utah)	0.001	0.005	0.012	0.029	0.054	0.089	0.132
Relative risk	4.0	4.0	2.75	2.79	3.78	5.93	4.0

*Modified from Meikle AW, Smith JA Jr, West DW: Familial factors affecting prostatic cancer risk and plasma sex steroid levels. *Prostate* 1985; 6:121–128. Used by permission.
†An overall fourfold increase in the probability of developing prostatic cancer is evident in brothers of patients with a known diagnosis of prostatic cancer compared with a general population of comparable age.

of prostatic cancer as well as benign prostatic diseases and the possible contribution of other factors make strong statements regarding possible associations difficult. However, there is no convincing evidence that a history of either bacterial or nonbacterial prostatitis or urethritis predisposes a patient to the development of carcinoma. Prostatic calculi are usually an incidental finding in patients with benign prostatic enlargement but have been reported in at least one study to occur with increased frequency in patients with prostatic cancer (Fig 1–2).[9]

There are conflicting data regarding the association of prostatic cancer and sexual practices. Some studies link sexual hyperactivity and promiscuity with an increased risk of prostatic cancer,[10, 11] while others suggest increased risk for those with repressed sexual activity,[12] including Catholic priests.[13] Similar confusion is apparent in reviewing the data regarding dietary factors in the development of prostatic cancer. It has been suggested by some that a high-fat diet contributes to carcinogenesis within the prostate, but this is unproven. There is no apparent association between cigarette smoking or alcohol intake and the development of carcinoma of the prostate.

The age at which prostatic cancer increases in frequency correlates with the development of benign prostatic hyperplasia. Therefore, it has been speculated that there may be an association between the two events. Approximately 10% of patients undergoing a transurethral prostatectomy for presumed benign prostatic hyperplasia are found to have microscopic adenocarcinoma.

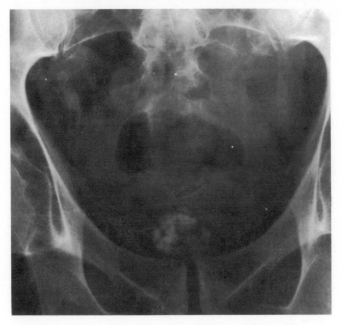

FIG 1–2.
Prostatic calculi visualized on plain film of pelvis. Prostate calculi are most commonly associated with benign prostatic hyperplasia rather than prostatic cancer.

However, the autopsy incidence of occult prostatic cancer in age-matched patients is similar. It seems likely that, despite the relatively common occurrence of prostatic cancer and benign enlargement in the same patient, etiologic factors for the two events are unrelated.

SYMPTOMS OF PROSTATIC CANCER

Knowledge of symptoms that may be associated with carcinoma of the prostate may help direct the clinician toward establishing the diagnosis and instituting appropriate therapy. Unfortunately, most localized prostatic cancers that are amenable to potentially curative therapy produce no symptoms. Locally advanced carcinoma of the prostate may cause symptoms of bladder outlet obstruction that mimic those seen in patients with benign prostatic hypertrophy. As the cancer enlarges, the flow of urine is restricted and patients may complain of hesitancy, dribbling, urinary frequency, nocturia, and a feeling of incomplete emptying. These symptoms may develop and progress more rapidly in patients with carcinoma of the prostate than in those with benign prostatic hyperplasia, but distinction between the two is not possible based simply upon symptoms and patient history. Sometimes, the voiding symptoms in patients with prostatic cancer are more related to rigidity within the prostatic capsule and bladder neck than to obstructive tissue alone. Hematuria, either gross or microscopic, may be seen occasionally in patients with prostatic cancer, but this is neither a sensitive nor a specific finding for the disease. Urinary tract infections may occur, especially if there is poor bladder emptying, but this also is a nonspecific finding. Independent of the effects of various treatments, there is generally no association between localized carcinoma of the prostate and sexual potency.

Patients with metastatic carcinoma of the prostate most often present with bone pain. Sometimes, especially in patients who have ignored bone pain or mistakenly attributed it to arthritis, a pathologic fracture or spinal cord compression is the presenting symptom. Cranial nerve palsies are seen occasionally in patients with basilar skull metastases. Lower-extremity edema may occur in situations where pelvic node metastases compromise venous return. Palpable lymph nodes, especially in the supraclavicular or inguinal region, may be the first sign of metastatic prostatic cancer. Soft-tissue metastases outside the lymphatic system are seen relatively frequently in patients with widespread skeletal metastases but are rarely the sole site of presentation of metastatic disease (Fig 1–3).

DIAGNOSIS OF PROSTATIC CANCER

Most often, the diagnosis of prostatic cancer is established because of a physical examination suggestive of the disease or signs and symptoms of metastatic tumor. The sensitivity and specificity of screening methods applied to the

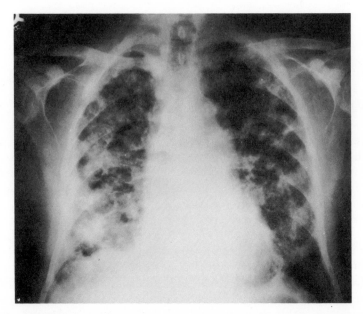

FIG 1–3.
Diffuse nodular and interstitial lung infiltrate from prostate cancer. Soft-tissue metastases of this extent are seen rarely without simultaneous bone involvement.

general population are insufficient for widespread application. Localized prostatic cancer is best detected by digital rectal examination, and it is recommended that this be performed on an annual basis in all men over the age of 50.

Prostatic Biopsy

Biopsy of the prostate is performed whenever there is a clinical suspicion of the presence of prostatic cancer. Usually, an area of induration, nodularity, or asymmetrical enlargement is detected on digital rectal examination. Sometimes, symptoms of distant metastatic disease have directed attention toward the prostate. In patients with metastatic adenocarcinoma of unknown primary, the prostate is sometimes considered as a source. However, in this setting, blind biopsy of a palpably normal prostate is unusually unrewarding.

By digital rectal palpation, a normal prostate gland is somewhat heart-shaped, with the base toward the bladder neck and the apex distally at the urogenital diaphragm (Fig 1–4). The base or superior aspect of the prostate is palpable as a transverse depression. Normal seminal vesicles are not palpable. The levator ani muscles are palpable at the lateral sulcus of the prostate. The normal consistency of the prostate is similar to that of the tip of the nose or the muscles of the thenar eminence of the hand; it is slightly compressible or spongy. Carcinoma of the prostate may be palpable as an area of nodularity that is raised from the surrounding surface of the prostate. Other times, the nodularity is less apparent but there is a loss of the usual planes surrounding the prostate at the lateral sulcus or base. Some degree of induration is almost always palpable. Often, only a deep induration is detectable rather than any irregularity or nodularity of the prostate.

Although a rectal examination may identify patients in whom there is a suspicion of adenocarcinoma of the prostate, other causes of prostatic induration and nodularity exist. Nodular forms of benign prostatic hypertrophy can occur resulting in irregular prostatic growth. Usually, these nodules are less indurated than those found in patients with carcinoma. Prostatitis or prostatic calculi can result in abnormal prostatic induration. An unusual form of prostatitis, granulomatous prostatitis, may be extremely difficult to distinguish from carcinoma by digital examination (Fig 1–5). Finally, postoperative changes and fibrosis, especially after a previous transurethral prostatectomy, can produce nodularity and induration difficult to distinguish from carcinoma.

The accuracy of a digital rectal examination as a screening test for carcinoma of the prostate is dependent upon the experience of the examiner and the frequency with which biopsy is recommended. However, prostatic biopsy should be performed whenever there is a palpable abnormality of the prostate that is suspicious of carcinoma if the patient is considered to be a candidate for therapy once the diagnosis is established. In general, this implies that there are some patients in whom biopsy may be deferred or, perhaps, not performed at all despite a clinical suspicion of prostatic cancer. Some elderly patients or those with significant medical problems may not be considered candidates for curative therapy by either surgery or irradiation. In these cir-

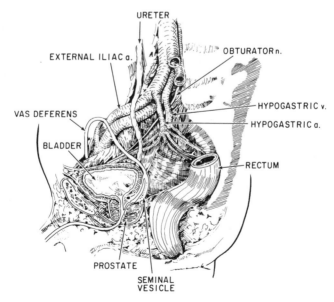

FIG 1–4.
Sagittal view of the pelvis showing the anatomical relationships of the prostate.

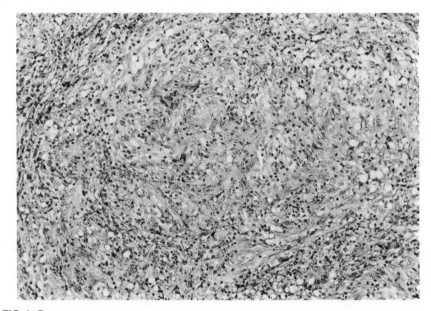

FIG 1–5.
Typical histologic findings of granulomatous prostatitis. Although the histologic changes are characteristic, physical examination may show an indurated lesion that cannot be distinguished from prostatic cancer.

cumstances, biopsy may be unnecessary and a needlessly invasive procedure if no immediate treatment is planned. The patient should be informed of the abnormality of the prostate and the possibility of carcinoma. If there is evidence of either local or distant disease progression, biopsy can be performed to confirm the diagnosis and appropriate palliative therapy instituted.

Once the decision has been made to perform a prostatic biopsy, a number of options are available. The decision regarding the type of biopsy should depend upon the experience and preference of the surgeon and pathologist as well as the size and location of the nodule.

Transperineal Biopsy

Core biopsies of the prostate can be obtained by placing a needle through the perineum into the suspicious area of the prostate (Fig 1–6). With a finger inserted into the rectum, the tip of the needle can be palpated and is directed into the suspicious area. Either a Vim-Silverman or a Tru-Cut needle is satisfactory for this purpose (Figs 1–7 and 1–8). The procedure can be performed with local infiltration of xylocaine into the perineum, but spinal or general anesthesia is often used.

Patients are placed in the lithotomy position. Often, prostate needle biopsy is preceded by cystoscopy for staging purposes (see chapter 2). An index finger is inserted into the rectum and the needle enters the perineum approxi-

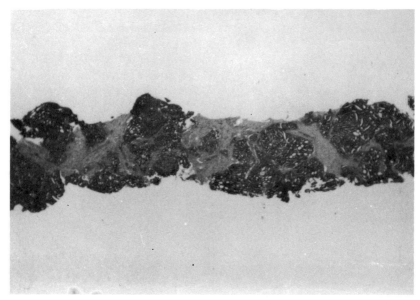

FIG 1–6.
Core of prostatic tissue obtained by perineal Tru-cut biopsy. The correlation between grading of material by histologic examination of core biopsies and cytologic interpretation of aspiration specimens has been excellent.

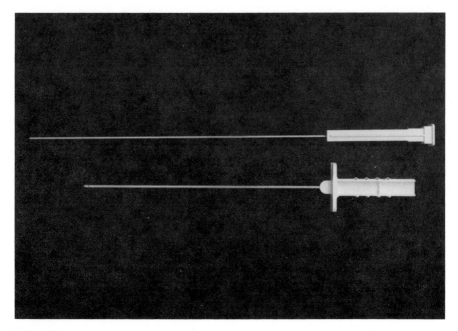

FIG 1–7.
Tru-cut needle for perineal biopsy of the prostate.

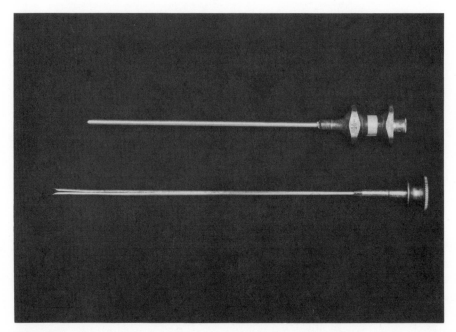

FIG 1–8.
Vim-Silverman needle for perineal biopsy of prostate. The cutting blades are inserted into the obturator, which is positioned within the suspicious portion of the prostate.

mately 2 cm above the anus. It is directed through the soft tissues of the perineum until the prostatic capsule is encountered. At this point, the tip of the needle is directed to the suspicious area and advanced. The obturator is withdrawn and the cutting blades of the Vim-Silverman needle are advanced into the suspicious area of the prostate. The sheath of the needle is then advanced over the cutting blades and twisted. The cutting blades are withdrawn and the core of prostatic tissue is removed and placed on a saline-soaked Telfa sponge. The mechanics of a Tru-Cut needle are similar to a Vim Silverman needle, but a Tru-Cut has the advantage of being a single piece that does not require interchanging of obturator and cutting blades. Prior to biopsy, it is not necessary to shave the skin of the perineum, although a sterile iodine-based skin preparation should be performed. A stab wound through the skin at the anticipated site of biopsy can be performed but is not necessary.

During the performance of transperineal prostatic biopsy, the tip of the needle may enter the bladder lumen. When the obturator or cutting blades are withdrawn from the biopsy needle, either urine or irrigating fluid from the cystoscopy drains through the biopsy needle. The needle is simply withdrawn and reinserted into the substance of the prostate. The number of cores of tissue that are taken is dependent upon the degree of suspicion, the size of the nodule, and the quality of the cores obtained. Especially if the patient is under an anesthetic, it seems a prudent policy to take multiple cores of the prostate to decrease the false-negative rate.

After the biopsy has been completed and a sufficient number of cores obtained, the needle is withdrawn from the perineum. Occasionally, some bleeding occurs from the skin wound, but this is easily controlled with local perineal pressure. A catheter should be inserted into the bladder to assess the amount of bleeding. If the urine is relatively clear and the patient does not have significant bladder outlet obstruction, the catheter can be removed. Occasionally, there is sufficient bleeding after prostate biopsy that it is advisable to leave a Foley catheter indwelling for several hours or overnight. Also, some patients experience enough edema or intraprostatic hemorrhage after biopsy that they develop urinary retention or difficulty voiding, and catheterization is required. More significant complications such as pelvic hemorrhage or sepsis are unusual. Routine antibiotics, either before or after transperineal biopsy of the prostate, are unnecessary. Implantation of tumor cells along the needle tract after prostatic biopsy is extremely uncommon but has been observed on occasion.

Transrectal Biopsy

As an alternative to transperineal biopsy, adequate cores of prostatic tissue can be obtained by the transrectal route. Proponents of this method claim greater ease in obtaining representative tissue from smaller nodules. Transrectal biopsy can be performed more easily under a local anesthetic than transperineal biopsy, but the incidence of complications is somewhat higher. Blood cultures are positive in over 80% of patients immediately after transrectal biopsy, although the incidence of bacteremia and clinically significant sepsis may be decreased with prebiopsy enemas of a 10% povidone-iodine solution. Broad-spectrum antibiotics should also be used. The most common organism causing infection after transrectal biopsy is *Escherichia coli*. Transrectal biopsy usually does not require an anesthetic.

The patient is placed in the lithotomy position and a Vim-Silverman or Tru-Cut needle is advanced into the rectum over the index finger. The abnormal area of the prostate is palpated and the needle advanced through the rectal wall into the substance of the prostate. Some discomfort is experienced by the patient when the needle is passed through the rectal wall. Multiple cores can be obtained by redirecting the needle. However, it is advisable not to withdraw the needle completely so that multiple punctures of the rectal wall are avoided.

Fine-Needle Aspiration

Fine-needle aspiration of the prostate can be a useful adjunct to core biopsy and, in some centers, has replaced it. The procedure does not require an anesthetic, and the incidence of postbiopsy bleeding and urinary retention is diminished. Furthermore, depending upon the method of fixation of the cellular specimen, the results can be available within hours. The primary disadvantage of aspiration biopsy of the prostate is the relative lack of experience with the procedure in this country as well as the need for an experienced cytopathologist to review the biopsies. Although the procedure is easy to learn, our studies have shown that the incidence of unsatisfactory specimens is proportionate to the experience of the surgeon performing the biopsy.[14]

Patients are placed in the lithotomy position. A Franzen needle guide is used for biopsy (Fig 1–9). This consists of a metal guide that is configured to the contour of the finger. The finger is placed into the rectum and a 22-gauge aspiration needle is inserted through the needle guide and directed through the rectal wall and into the substance of the prostate. A 10-cc syringe is used to apply suction to the needle tip, which is moved successively throughout the substance of the prostate gland. There often appears to be little or no tissue aspirated from the prostate but, if performed properly, there is abundant cellular material obtained (Fig 1–10). This is ejected onto a clean glass slide and then fixed and stained with appropriate solution. Antibiotics have not been used as a routine after aspiration biopsy.

In the hands of an experienced cytopathologist, the false-positive rate for aspiration biopsy of the prostate should be extremely low. The false-positive cases that have been described generally are reported as such because core

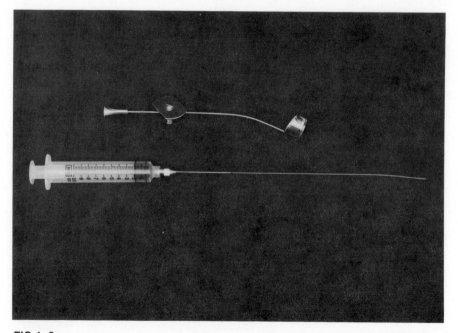

FIG 1–9.
Modified Franzen needles for aspiration biopsy of the prostate. The thin needle is inserted transrectally into the suspicious area of the prostate. Suction on the syringe is used to obtain cellular material.

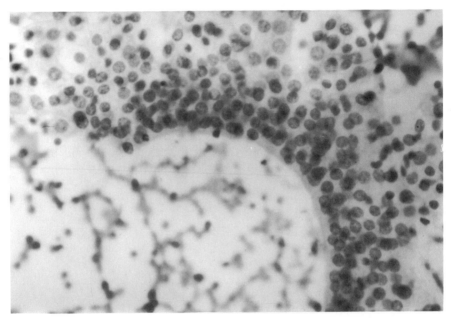

FIG 1–10.
Normal prostatic cells obtained by transrectal needle aspiration. Abundant cellular material can be obtained by needle aspiration.

biopsy failed to confirm the diagnosis. In Scandinavia, where the technique has gained great popularity, false-negative rates with transrectal aspiration biopsy are no lower than those seen with core biopsy. However, in most centers with less experience, the false-negative rate of aspiration biopsy is somewhat higher.

A problem that arises is how to interpret a positive aspiration biopsy that cannot be confirmed by a core biopsy (Fig 1–11). The approximate 10% false-negative rate with core biopsy opens the possibility that the aspiration biopsy is correct rather than a false-positive under these circumstances. Our flow chart for the use of aspiration biopsy and the clinical interpretation of its results is depicted in Figure 1–12. In general, a positive aspiration biopsy for moderately or poorly differentiated carcinoma is considered diagnostic of prostatic cancer (Fig 1–13). If the aspiration shows well-differentiated cells, confirmation of cancer is performed by needle biopsy (Fig 1–14). Finally, if aspiration biopsy is negative but a clinically suspicious nodule is present, needle biopsy is performed.

Histologic Types of Prostatic Cancer

The overwhelming majority of prostatic cancers are adenocarcinomas that arise from the epithelium of the prostatic acini, usually in the periphery of the

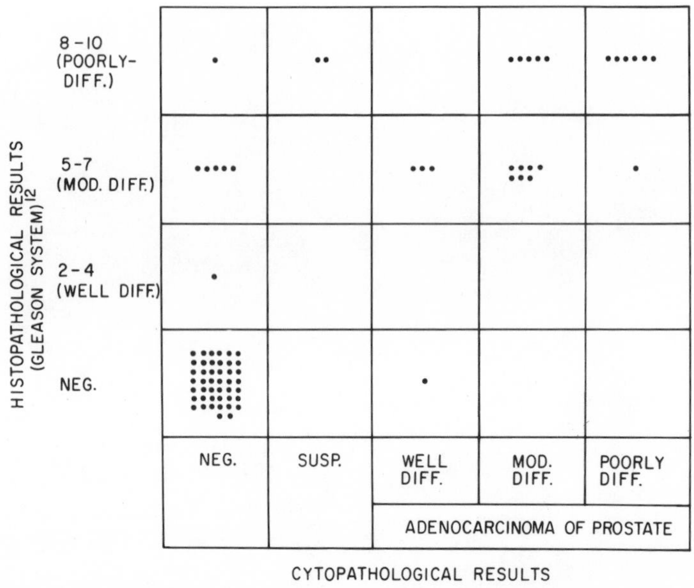

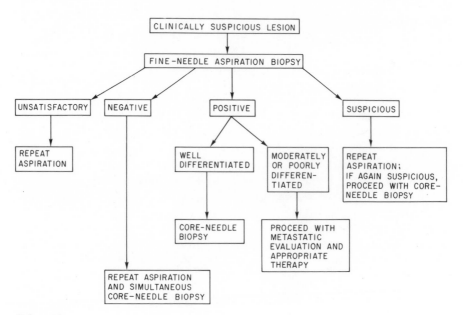

FIG 1–11.
Chart showing the correlation between histopathologic results after needle biopsy of the prostate and cytologic results after aspiration in patients with prostate nodules. A similar correlation has been observed in a number of other studies.

FIG 1–12.
Flow diagram for use of fine-needle aspiration of the prostate.

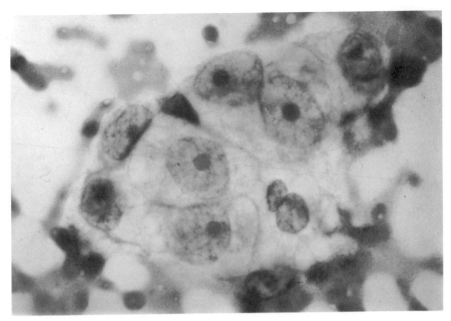

FIG 1–13.
Cells consistent with poorly differentiated adenocarcinoma obtained by fine-needle aspiration of the prostate.

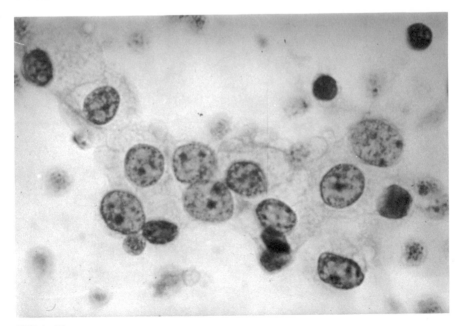

FIG 1–14.
Cells consistent with well-differentiated adenocarcinoma obtained by needle aspiration of the prostate. False-positive errors are possible with well-differentiated cells, and a confirmatory core biopsy of the prostate often is necessary before definitive therapy is undertaken.

prostate gland. Primary transitional cell carcinomas of the prostate can occur and usually originate from the prostatic periurethral ducts. In addition, intra-ductal adenocarcinomas have been described. They are thought to have less androgen dependence than acinar adenocarcinoma and may have a worse overall prognosis, but treatment considerations are the same. Even less com-mon are sarcomas, usually of smooth muscle (leiomyosarcoma) or, especially in children, skeletal muscle (rhabdomyosarcoma) (Fig 1–15). The prostate gland is rarely the site of metastatic tumors. Although bladder cancers may directly invade the substance of the prostate, Dennonvilier's fascia usually forms an effective barrier limiting direct extension between the prostate gland and adjacent rectal carcinomas. Lymphocytic or leukemic infiltrates of the prostate are sometimes seen in patients with lymphoma or leukemia and generally form a diffuse, symmetric but indurated enlargement of the prostate (Fig 1–16).

Another histologic cell type of carcinoma that has been described is en-dometrioid carcinoma of the prostate. Since these tumors have a histologic appearance similar to endometrioid carcinoma in women, it has been postu-lated that they arise from the residual Müllerian duct tissue of the prostatic utricle.[15] In addition, there were earlier suggestions that estrogen therapy was contraindicated with this tumor.[16] More recent evidence has cast doubt upon the origin of endometrioid tumors and has suggested that these tumors re-spond in a similar fashion as prostatic ductile carcinoma to hormonal therapy.

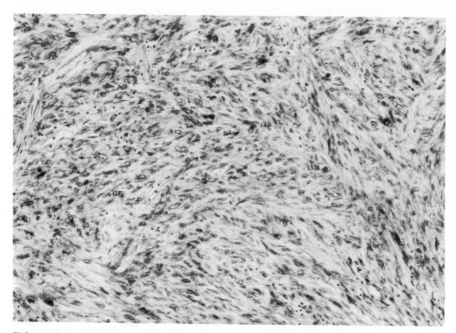

FIG 1–15.
Poorly differentiated sarcoma of the prostate. Although relatively uncommon, sarcomatous lesions of the prostate usually have a more spongy consistency than adenocarcinoma.

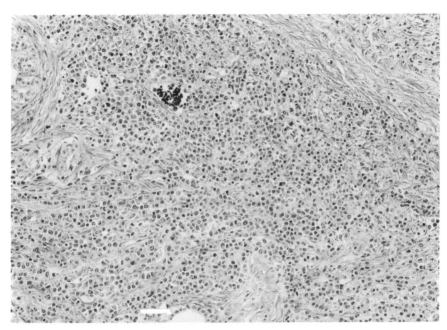

FIG 1–16.
Leukemic infiltration of prostate. The prostate gland is a rare site of metastasis from other tumors, but diffuse infiltration by lymphoma or leukemia is sometimes observed.

Although these tumors may behave in a somewhat more indolent fashion than other prostatic cancers, stage for stage treatment options generally are the same as for acinar adenocarcinoma.

GRADING

Grading of prostatic adenocarcinoma has been shown to be of prognostic significance and may have implications regarding choice of therapy. A diagnosis of adenocarcinoma of the prostate is based upon several alterations in the normal histologic appearance of the prostate. The size or configuration of prostatic acini is altered to some degree in prostatic cancers. Tumors that more closely resemble the normal prostatic glandular pattern are considered better differentiated than those that cause severe disfigurement or loss of the glandular pattern. Well-differentiated tumors frequently consist of small, densely packed glands, whereas poorly differentiated tumors may lose all gross architectural integrity and appear as sheets of cells with little tendency to form glands (Figs 1–17 through 1–19).

The internal architecture of the prostatic acini also may be disturbed in prostatic cancer. Normally, a double layer of columnar cells is seen in prostatic

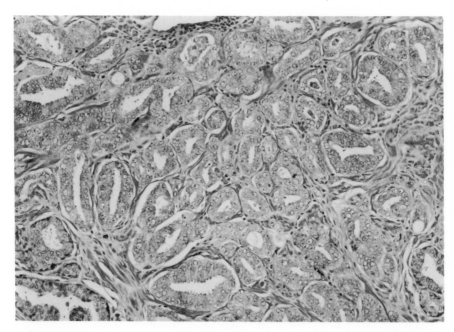

FIG 1–17.
Well-differentiated adenocarcinoma of the prostate. Closely packed glands with single cell layers are evident.

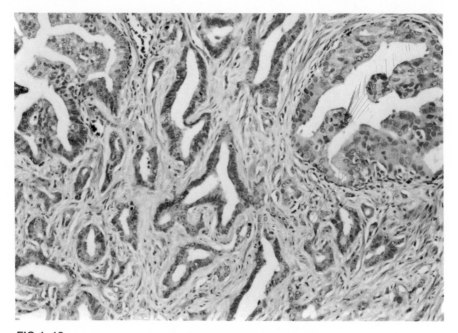

FIG 1–18.
Moderately differentiated adenocarcinoma of the prostate.

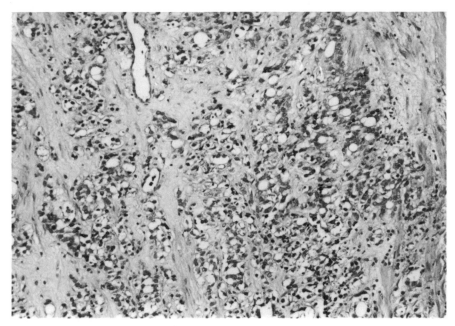

FIG 1–19.
Poorly differentiated adenocarcinoma of the prostate. Sheets of cells are seen with little tendency for gland formation.

acini. In malignant lesions, there is usually only a single layer of low cuboidal cells. A characteristic cribriform pattern may also appear (Fig 1–20).

Another consideration sometimes used in grading prostatic cancer is the appearance of the individual cells, that is, the degree of anaplasia. As with other tumors, malignant prostatic cancer cells may show pleomorphism and an increased nuclear/cytoplasmic ratio. The nuclei may appear hyperchromatic and be variable in size and shape. Mitotic figures usually are not seen.

Currently, most grading systems for prostatic cancer utilize one or all of the above parameters to determine the tumor grade. The Mostofi system takes into consideration not only the gross glandular architecture, but also the individual cellular characteristics.[17] Grade I tumors are those in which gland formation is retained and individual cellular anaplasia is slight. Gland formation may also be preserved in grade II tumors, but nuclear anaplasia is more pronounced. A tumor may be considered grade III based upon either the absence of gland formation or marked nuclear anaplasia.

The Gleason grading system was used initially by the Veterans Administration Cooperative Urologic Research Group in the 1960s.[18] With this system, individual cellular characteristics are not considered. Rather, under low-power magnification, the degree of glandular differentiation and the relationship of the glands to the prostatic stroma are evaluated. Tumors are graded from 1 to 5 (from the most well differentiated to the most anaplastic). Many tumors ex-

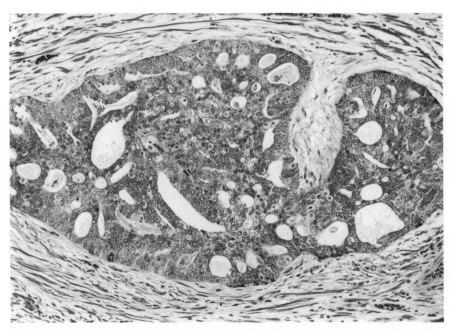

FIG 1–20.
Typical cribiform pattern of moderately differentiated prostatic cancer.

hibit two primary histologic patterns. Therefore, to accommodate these variabilities, the system includes both a primary and a secondary Gleason grade with the total Gleason score representing the sum of the two. Accordingly, histologic scores range from 2 to 10.

Other prostatic cancer grading systems have evolved.[19, 20] Nevertheless, despite subtle differences between the various systems, each generally appears to group biopsy specimens similarly. Therefore, tumors that are considered low grade or well differentiated by one system frequently fall into the same category by another. Likewise, the most poorly differentiated and, presumably, more virulent tumors are similarly identified by each grading system. There is variability in the reproduction of grading between pathologists and even variability by the same pathologist. However, these differences are usually relatively slight, and most biopsy specimens fall generally within the same categories (well differentiated, moderately undifferentiated, and poorly differentiated) despite the system of grading used or the pathologist.

Cytology

Assignment of tumor grade is also possible based on cytologic specimens obtained by aspiration. Well-differentiated tumors tend to display less pleomorphism and nuclear anaplasia and are also seen as clumps of cells. On the other hand, poorly differentiated lesions often are seen as individual cells with marked nuclear anaplasia and prominent nucleoli. Correlation between cytologic and histologic grade may be variable but, for practical clinical purposes, the tumors that are poorly differentiated and have an unfavorable prognosis are readily distinguished from those with well-differentiated histologic characteristics and presumably a more indolent course. Cytologic examination of voided urine specimens usually is unrewarding and its sensitivity is insufficient to make it a useful clinical tool.

Immunofluorescence and Acid Phosphatase Staining

The usefulness of serum acid phosphatase determinations by enzymatic or radioimmunoassay techniques in staging prostatic cancer is discussed in chapter 2. However, acid phosphatase staining can also be used to help identify the prostate as the site of origin of a poorly differentiated tumor at the bladder neck or a metastatic carcinoma of unknown primary. Prostatic acid phosphatase is contained within secretory granules of prostatic epithelial cells. Prostatic acid phosphatase is a sensitive but not a specific marker for prostatic cancer. Thus, the presence of acid phosphatase within a cancer cell is insufficient evidence to establish definitively the prostate as the primary site. Prostatic acid phosphatase has been found in pancreatic tumors, in some breast carcinomas, and in up to two thirds of rectal carcinoid tumors.[21]

Prostate-Specific Antigen

A human prostate-specific antigen was reported in 1979.[22] Prostate-specific antigen (PSA) can be an effective immunohistologic marker for prostatic cancer. It is of use in the differential diagnosis of metastatic carcinomas of unknown primary origin or in distinguishing poorly differentiated prostatic cancer invading the bladder neck or trigone from transitional cell carcinoma.[23] The PSA level is elevated in the substantial majority of patients with metastatic prostatic cancer and may be abnormal in some with intracapsular disease.[24] Although PSA appears to be the most sensitive and specific marker for prostatic cancer yet defined, it is unlikely to be useful as a screening test for segments of a general population.

REFERENCES

1. Cancer statistics, 1986. *Ca* 1986; 36:16–17.
2. Holund B: Latent prostatic cancer in a consecutive autopsy series. *Scand J Urol Nephrol* 1982; 42:3864–3869.
3. Murphy GP, Natarajan N, Pontes JE, et al: The National Survey of Prostate Cancer in the United States by the American College of Surgeons. *J Urol* 1982; 127:928–934.
4. Hutchison GB: Epidemiology of prostatic cancer. *Semin Oncol* 1976; 3:151–159.

5. Jackson MA, Ahluwalia BS, Herson J, et al: Characterization of prostatic carcinoma among blacks: A continuation report. *Cancer Treat Rep* 1977; 61:167–172.
6. Winkelstein W Jr, Ernster VL: Epidemiology and etiology, in Murphy GP (ed): *Prostatic Cancer*. Littleton, Mass, PSG Publishing Co, 1979, pp 1–17.
7. Yantani R, Chigusa I, Akazaki K, et al: Geographic pathology of latent prostatic carcinoma. *Int J Cancer* 1982; 29:611–616.
8. Meikle AW, Smith JA Jr, West DW: Familial factors affecting prostatic cancer risk and plasma sex steroid levels. *Prostate* 1985; 6:121–128.
9. Ioachim H: La lithiase prostitique peut-elle etre consideree comme un facteur cancerogene? *Urologia* 1961; 28:1–12.
10. Schuman LM, Mandel J, Blackard C, et al: Epidemiologic study of prostatic cancer: Preliminary report. *Cancer Treat Rep* 1977; 61:181–186.
11. Steele R, Lees REM, Kraus AS, et al: Sexual factors in the epidemiology of cancer of the prostate. *J Chronic Dis* 1971; 24:29–37.
12. Rotkin ID: Studies in the epidemiology of prostatic cancer: Expanded sampling. *Cancer Treat Rep* 1977; 61:173–180.
13. Ross RK, McCurtis JW, Henderson BE, et al: Descriptive epidemiology of testicular and prostatic cancer in Los Angeles. *Br J Cancer* 1979; 39:284–292.
14. Wood TS, Debellis C, Schumann B, et al: Fine-needle aspiration of the prostate, in preparation.
15. Melicow MM, Pachter MR: Endometrial carcinoma of prostatic utricle (uterus masculinus). *Cancer* 1967; 20:1715–1722.
16. Melicow MM, Tannenbaum M: Endometrial carcinoma of uterus masculinus (prostatic utricle): Report of 6 cases. *J Urol* 1971; 106:892–902.
17. Mostofi FK: Problems of grading carcinoma of prostate. *Semin Oncol* 1976; 3: 161–169.
18. Gleason DF: Classification of prostatic carcinomas. *Cancer Chemother Rep* 1966; 50:125–128.
19. Gaeta JF, Asirwatham JE, Miller G, et al: Histologic grading of primary prostatic cancer: A new approach to an old problem. *J Urol* 1980; 123:689–693.
20. Utz DC, Farrow GM: Pathologic differentiation and prognosis of prostatic carcinoma. *JAMA* 1969; 209:1701–1703.
21. Sobin PAP activity in carcinoid tumors. *Cancer* 1986; 1:135–138.
22. Wang MC, Valenzuala LA, Murphy GP, et al: Purification of a human prostate specific antigen. *Invest Urol* 1979; 17:159–163.
23. Ming Chu T, Murphy GP: What's new in tumor markers for prostate cancer? *Urology* 1986; 27:487–491.
24. Tumor markers in the follow-up of initial therapy of prostatic cancer, in Lange PH (ed): *Tumor Markers in Prostatic Cancer*. Princeton, NJ, Excerpta Medica, 1986, pp 16–23.

2

Staging of Prostate Cancer

Staging of prostatic cancer involves determination of the size and local extent of the tumor as well as detection of distant foci either in lymphatics, bone, or soft tissue. Although accurate staging is a necessary part of evaluation of any tumor, it is of even greater importance in prostatic cancer, a disease in which aggressive local therapy may not be indicated for all patients. In some patients, tumors that are detected at an early, localized stage have a sufficiently slow progression rate that aggressive therapy with curative intent may not be justified. On the other hand, local tumor progression in these patients or the finding of metastatic disease may be an indication for therapy.

Selection of therapy for patients with prostatic cancer is directly dependent upon stage of the tumor. While those with a sufficiently long life expectancy and localized disease should be offered aggressive therapy with curative intent, patients with metastatic disease or advanced local lesions are unlikely to benefit from such treatment and should be spared the morbidity of therapy.

Various staging classifications for prostatic cancer have been described, but the one proposed by Whitmore and modified by Jewett has endured as one that sufficiently categorizes patients for treatment purposes (Table 2–1). Under this classification system, patients are divided into various categories designated by a letter and a numerical subset. Another commonly used staging system is that proposed by the Union Internationale Contre Le Cancer (UICC), sometimes called the TNM system. The TNM system uses the T category to define the extent of the primary tumor, the N to describe lymph node status, and the M to indicate distant metastases. As such, it is a more complete and descriptive staging system than the commonly used Whitmore-Jewett classification. However, because of its widespread acceptance, the Jewett modification of the Whitmore system is used throughout this book.

Subsequent chapters deal extensively with the treatment options for the various stages of prostatic cancer. However, a brief description of the stages follows:

TABLE 2–1.

Staging of Prostatic Cancer

WHITMORE–JEWETT SYSTEM	UICC	DESCRIPTION
A1	T0a	Microscopic focal tumors, generally fewer than 5 foci or less than 5% area
A2	T0b	Microscopic but diffuse cancer; includes all high-grade microscopic tumors
B1	T1a, T1b	Palpable nodule <2 cm in size or confined to one lobe of prostate
B2	T1c, T2	Palpable nodule >2 cm in size or involving both lobes of prostate
C	T3, T4	Palpable tumor that extends beyond prostatic capsule to involve seminal vesicles or lateral pelvic wall
D0	T0–T4, N−,M−	Elevated acid phosphatase level, without other evidence of disease beyond prostate or periprostate region
D1	T0–T4, N+, M−	Lymph node metastasis without evident extrapelvic disease
D2	T0–T4, N+, M+	Metastatic disease outside the pelvis, usually to bone

Stage A.—Stage A adenocarcinoma of the prostate is defined as tumor detected upon histologic examination of a prostatectomy specimen when the procedure was performed for presumed benign prostatic hyperplasia. Thus, although often considered a clinical stage, it is by definition a pathologic diagnosis. Because of marked differences in prognosis and, therefore, treatment implications, stage A prostatic cancer is further subdivided into stage A1 and stage A2.

Stage A1 (UICC Stage T0a).—Various criteria are used to define stage A1 carcinoma of the prostate. In general, the foci of microscopic carcinoma are quantified either numerically or as a percentage of the total prostatic tissue. We have used five or fewer foci of carcinoma as the criterion for stage A1 carcinoma of the prostate, but other classifications have described A1 as tumor involvement of less than 5% of the total prostatic tissue resected or enucleated.[2] A1 carcinoma of the prostate is generally considered to be an incidental finding and is unlikely to be of clinical significance. High-grade tumors are often excluded from this category regardless of the total number of foci or percent involvement.

Stage A2 (UICC Stage T0b).—More than five foci of microscopic adenocarcinoma or more than 5% total involvement of the specimen with prostatic cancer is considered stage A2. Also, all high-grade carcinomas identified in the surgical specimen of patients undergoing prostatectomy for presumed benign prostatic hyperplasia should be considered stage A2.

Stage B.—Stage B carcinoma of the prostate is defined as a palpable nodule or area of induration that apparently is confined within the capsule of the prostate gland.

Stage B1 (UICC Stage T1a or T1b).—The classic stage B1 adenocarcinoma of the prostate is described by Jewett[1] as a nodule of less than 1½ cm in size that is surrounded by palpably normal prostatic tissue. Currently, most urologists would broaden this category somewhat and include small nodules located at the periphery of the prostate if they seem to be palpably confined within the capsule and are less than 2 cm in size.

Stage B2 (UICC Stage T1c or T2).—A palpable nodule that exceeds 2 cm in size but still seems to be confined within the capsule of the prostate is considered stage B2 adenocarcinoma. Also included in this category would be patients with two distinct areas of nodularity even though both may be less than 2 cm in size.

Stage C.—Stage C prostatic cancers are those that have not metastasized to distant areas or lymph nodes, but that locally have extended beyond the confines of the prostatic capsule. Most commonly, stage C tumors extend laterally into the levator muscles of the pelvic side wall or superiorly into the seminal vesicles and bladder base.

Stage C1 (UICC Stage T3).—Stage C1 includes tumors with minimal amounts of palpable extracapsular extension.

Stage C2 (UICC Stage T_4).—Stage C2 tumors are large (greater than 5 cm) and may cause symptomatic bladder outlet or ureteral obstruction.

Stage D.—Stage D tumors are those that have metastasized beyond the periprostatic region.

Stage D0.—This category is designed to include patients in whom the only evidence of metastatic disease is an elevated serum acid phosphatase level.

Stage D1 (UICC T0–T4, N+).—Stage D1 tumors are those that have spread to involve the pelvic lymph nodes but are not detected in any other distant site. By the Whitmore-Jewett system, the extent of the primary tumor is irrelevant in defining stage if nodes are positive. In the UICC system, the size and extent of the primary tumor is defined under the T category.

Stage D2 (UICC T0–T4, N+, M+).—This category encompasses prostatic tumors that have metastasized beyond the pelvic lymph nodes. Stage D2 usually identifies patients with bone metastases, but it also includes those with soft-tissue metastases and lymph node involvement outside the pelvis.

STAGING LOCAL EXTENT

Determining the degree of local spread of a prostatic cancer is critical in selecting patients for appropriate therapy. The most important distinction is whether the tumor is contained within the capsule of the prostate gland (stage A or B) or whether there is extracapsular extension (stage C). Not only is there a prognostic difference between the two groups, but certain treatments or surgical procedures that may be appropriate for one category are not applicable to others. The most obvious example is the selection of patients for radical prostatectomy. Most urologic surgeons feel that patients with stage B and, perhaps, stage A tumors are appropriate candidates for a radical prostatectomy, while those with stage C lesions have tumors that cannot be totally excised surgically. Therefore, if there is no evidence of distant metastatic disease, determination of local extent of the tumor becomes extremely important. Various procedures may be useful in determining the presence or absence of capsular invasion, seminal vesicle involvement, or both.

Digital Palpation

The simplest and least costly method for determining the local extent of prostatic cancer, digital palpation, is also the one that provides the most information.[3] Not all prostatic cancers are palpable. Indeed, stage A tumors are those that, by definition, are not detected by digital palpation of the prostate prior to a prostatectomy. However, most clinically significant tumors are evident as an area of induration or nodularity within the prostate.

Overstaging in prostatic cancer rarely occurs clinically, although periprostatic bleeding shortly after a biopsy of the prostate may obscure tissue planes. On the other hand, understaging is a more important issue. In historical series, the incidence of understaging of stage B tumors is significant. Seminal vesicle involvement or extracapsular extension has been noted in as many as 15% to 20% of patients with clinical stage B1 tumors and up to half of those who clinically were thought to have stage B2 lesions.[4] Thus, the accuracy of digital palpation of the prostate alone as a means of staging local extent of prostatic cancer has been questioned. Undoubtedly, other factors should be considered, and the status of the pelvic lymph nodes has been found to be somewhat predictive of local tumor extent.[5] Nevertheless, careful digital examination of the prostate remains the most important staging maneuver in apparently localized prostatic cancer and the standard by which other methods must be compared. Bimanual examination of the prostate with the patient under an anesthetic may provide more accurate staging information but is not mandatory in all patients.

Cystourethroscopy

Endoscopic examination of the prostatic urethra and bladder neck should be performed in all patients with localized prostatic cancer. Since carcinoma of the prostate most often arises in the peripheral portion of the gland, cystoscopy findings are frequently normal with relatively small tumors. However, tumor invasion of the bladder neck or the trigone may be detected at cystoscopy, thus altering the prognosis and treatment options. Also, the degree of bladder outlet obstruction and bladder trabeculation should be assessed. Endoscopically, the lateral lobes of the prostate are usually symmetric unless the tumor is extensive.

Intravenous Pyelography

Intravenous (IV) pyelography traditionally has been a standard staging maneuver in patients with prostatic cancer and may provide information that is otherwise not obtainable. Ureteral obstruction may be seen with large, local lesions due to tumor infiltration of the bladder base (Fig 2–1). Also, enlarged pelvic lymph nodes can produce deviation of the course of the pelvic ureter

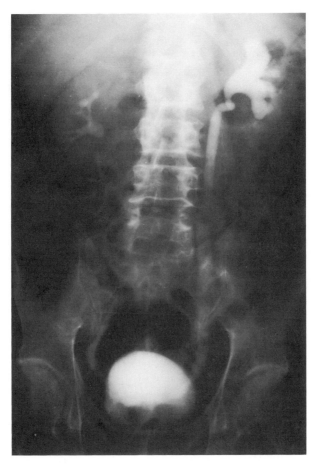

FIG 2–1.
Obstruction of left distal ureter from local extension of prostate cancer.

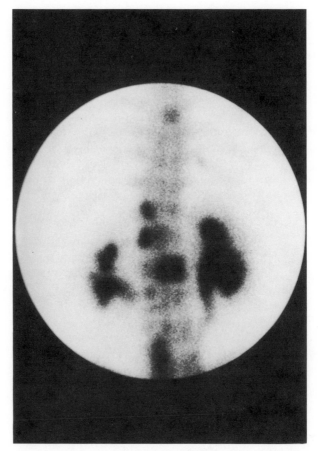

FIG 2–2.
Bone scan showing several areas of metastatic uptake in lumbar spine. In addition, bilateral retention of the radionuclide in the kidneys is evident secondary to ureteral obstruction. Although a bone scan gives relatively imprecise anatomical detail, it can be useful in excluding or detecting obstructing uropathy.

or obstruction of the ureter at the pelvic brim. If other studies, such as computed tomographic (CT) scanning or ultrasonography have been obtained and have shown no evidence of hydronephrosis, IV pyelography may not be necessary in all patients with prostatic cancer. In addition, nuclear bone scans can give a gross assessment of ureteral obstruction, although the architectural detail is less than that obtained with pyelography (Fig 2–2).

Ultrasonography

Ultrasonography of the kidneys can be obtained to rule out hydronephrosis in patients with prostatic cancer. Of greater interest, however, has been transrectal ultrasonic examination of the prostate to assist in determining the local extent of the tumor. Normally, the prostate gland produces a diffuse echo pattern, with a similar finding being seen in patients with benign prostatic hyperplasia. Carcinoma of the prostate may produce dense echos that can be distinguished from the normal-appearing prostate. In addition, there is often an irregular appearance to the echo-dense area and there may be deformity in the prostatic capsule. Anechoic or hypoechoic lesions in the peripheral portion of the prostate are also frequently indicative of prostatic cancer. Areas of prostatitis or prostatic calculi may be difficult to distinguish from carcinoma.

Transrectal ultrasonography has been used in an attempt to detect clinically occult carcinoma (stage A). The lack of specificity of the procedure has made it ineffective as a screening device for an asymptomatic population.[6] Lee and colleagues[7] have used transrectal ultrasonography to screen patients, but the superiority of this method over rectal examination has not been demonstrated.[7] Of 55 men with a palpably normal prostate but abnormal transrectal ultrasonographic findings, Cohen and Resnick[8] found only nine to have adenocarcinoma. Occasional false-negative examination results were found in patients with diffusely infiltrating tumors which obscured tissue interfaces.

In patients with known, palpable tumors, transrectal ultrasonography has been investigated as a means of detecting nonpalpable extracapsular tumor spread. Scardino et al.[9] found that ultrasonography accurately identified extracapsular extension in 45 (83%) of 54 patients undergoing radical prostatectomy who had been thought to have stage A or B tumors on rectal examination. Ultrasonography incorrectly predicted extracapsular spread in 27% of patients with histologically proven localized tumors.[9] The accuracy of ultrasonography as an adjunct to rectal examination in detecting extracapsular tumor extension remains undetermined and must be tested on a widespread clinical basis.

Computed Tomography

Computed tomography scanning of the prostate has been disappointing and relatively inaccurate in staging local extent of prostatic cancer. In certain projections, CT images through the prostate can provide fairly accurate anatomical information regarding the relationship between the bladder, prostate, and seminal vesicles (Fig 2–3). However, the configuration and location of the prostate deep within the pelvis create difficulty with visualization. The curved planes surrounding the prostate are not well displayed on transverse cuts with CT scanning, and horizontal projections may be confusing. Computed tomographic scanning is relatively nonspecific, and irregularity or enlargement within the prostate gland is difficult to interpret. Overstaging may occur with CT scanning, especially after biopsy or other procedures that produce bleeding or edema within or around the prostate.

Magnetic Resonance Imaging of the Prostate

Magnetic resonance imaging (MRI) of the pelvis and prostate has been professed to be a more accurate means for potential staging of prostatic cancer

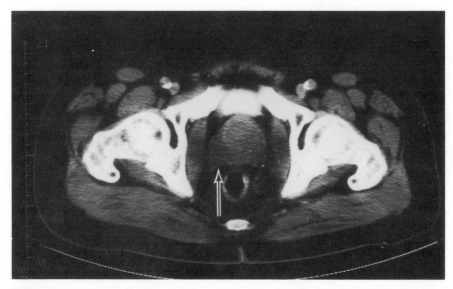

FIG 2–3.
Extracapsular tumor extension from prostatic cancer visualized by CT scan. Overall, CT scanning has not been particularly useful in staging local extent of prostatic cancer.

than CT scanning.[10] A more refined image is obtained and the prostatic capsule and seminal vesicles frequently are readily visible (Fig 2–4). Although the procedure seems promising, the accuracy of MRI in staging prostatic cancer is undetermined. Furthermore, as with CT scanning, abnormalities within the prostate are relatively nonspecific, and postbiopsy changes may result in overstaging of some tumors.

LYMPH NODE STAGING

The first echelon of metastasis beyond the prostate is usually the pelvic lymph nodes. Obviously, in a situation wherein extrapelvic metastases are evident, the status of the pelvic lymph nodes becomes unimportant. However, when definitive local therapy is being contemplated for an otherwise localized prostatic cancer, detection of pelvic lymph node metastasis becomes critical since this may alter treatment plans or intent.

A number of potential methods for evaluation of the pelvic lymph nodes have been described. To some extent, the method chosen depends on the stage of the primary tumor and the manner in which the information obtained is used. Noninvasive staging techniques such as CT scanning or lymphangiography may be more useful in higher stage or grade tumors wherein gross nodal metastases may occur. On the other hand, if whole pelvic irradiation is the planned therapy, a surgical lymphadenectomy may be inadvisable since lower extremity edema may result from the combination of lymphadenectomy and irradiation. Each of the potential methods for evaluating the pelvic lymph nodes is discussed along with the advantages and disadvantages of each.

Lymphangiography

Lymphangiography has often been mentioned and used as a method to evaluate the pelvic lymph nodes in patients with prostatic cancer. The technique involves injection of Lipiodol into lymphatic vessels on the dorsum of the feet. The radiographic substance migrates through the lymphatics of the legs, and radiographs 24 hours after injections show filling of the pelvic lymph nodes. An abnormal study occurs when filling defects within the lymph nodes are identified or when there is gross distortion of the architecture of the lymph node (Fig 2–5). Controversy persists regarding whether or not the lymph nodes that represent the primary drainage of the prostate are consistently filled on pedal lymphangiograms.[10] Part of the problem resides in semantics. Traditionally, surgeons have referred to the obturator lymph nodes as the primary drainage of the prostate although this lymph node group frequently includes

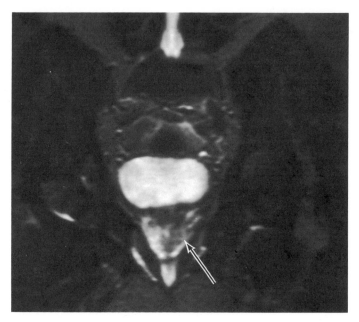

FIG 2–4.
T_2 weighted (TR 2500, TE 80) MRI scan showing extracapsular extension of prostatic cancer. Magnetic resonance imaging provides relatively well-defined anatomical detail of the prostate, but its role in staging prostate cancer is unclear.

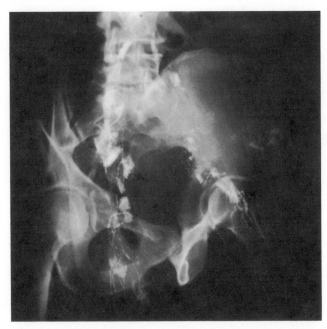

FIG 2–5.
Tumor metastasis to right pelvic lymph nodes. Lymphangiography may be useful in detecting pelvic node metastasis in patients with high-grade, large-volume primary tumors wherein gross nodal metastases may be evident.

medial portions of the external iliac drainage as well as some of the hypogastric lymph nodes.

False-positive interpretation of lymphangiograms is unacceptable since a positive study result may drastically alter therapy or, perhaps, remove a patient from consideration of definitive treatment. Using strict criteria of interpretation decreases the false-positive rate to around 10%, although inflammation, fatty infiltration, or benign lymphoid hyperplasia may create confusion. In general, a lymphangiogram should not be accepted as positive without histologic confirmation by fine-needle aspiration (Fig 2–6).

The primary limitation of lymphangiography in staging prostatic cancer is an inordinately high false-negative rate. Only around one fourth of patients with histologically proven lymph node metastases have preoperative identification of lymph node metastases on lymphangiography.[11] Extensive metastatic disease that completely replaces a lymph node may result in nonfilling and lack of detection by lymphangiography (Fig 2–7). More commonly, only microscopic involvement of lymph nodes is present which does not distort the internal architecture of the lymph node. Thus, lymphangiography is a relatively insensitive method for detecting pelvic lymph node metastasis compared to lymphadenectomy. Furthermore, lymphangiography is not completely without morbidity.

Ultrasonography

Ultrasonography is capable of detecting gross lymph node metastases which result in enlargement of lymph nodes to greater than 2 cm. Usually, lymph node enlargement to this degree does not occur in the absence of distant metastatic disease. Therefore, ultrasonography is an insensitive technique for staging pelvic lymph nodes.

Computed Tomographic Scanning

Computed tomographic scanning of the pelvis is another noninvasive yet relatively insensitive method for staging pelvic lymph nodes in patients with prostatic cancer (Fig 2–8). Although CT scanning cannot detect microscopic disease, it can identify lymph nodes of greater than 1.5 cm in size. Benign enlargement or hyperplasia may exceed that figure, so fine-needle aspiration is necessary to eliminate false-positive results (Fig 2–9). Unopacified loops of bowel may also present confusion as well as confluent blood vessels.

Despite these limitations, CT scanning is probably the preferred method for noninvasive staging of prostatic cancer. The sensitivity exceeds ultrasonography and approaches that of lymphangiography, and there is no morbidity associated with the procedure.[12] In general, it should be recognized that only about half of the patients with histologic pelvic node metastases will be identified by pelvic CT scanning. However, the procedure may be useful in selected patients with higher grade tumors wherein gross nodal metastasis is more common.

Magnetic Resonance Imaging

Magnetic resonance imaging can provide detailed displays of pelvic anatomy. However, the technique is subject to the same limitations as CT scanning in that minimal pelvic lymph node enlargement or microscopic metastases cannot be detected. The superiority of MRI over CT scanning of the pelvis as a means of staging pelvic lymph nodes has not been demonstrated.

Fine-Needle Aspiration

In all patients selected for noninvasive staging of pelvic nodes, fine-needle aspiration should be performed to histologically confirm a positive study[13] (Fig 2–10). Fine-needle aspiration can be used as an adjunct to any of the procedures mentioned above. A 22-gauge needle is directed to the abnormal lymph node or area of lymph node identified, and aspiration should yield cellular material for microscopic examination. Abnormal lymph nodes identified on lymphangiography, ultrasonography, CT scanning, or MRI should be punctured and an aspiration performed.

Use of fine-needle aspiration as an adjunct to these staging procedures should eliminate false-positive errors. However, the technique does not rule

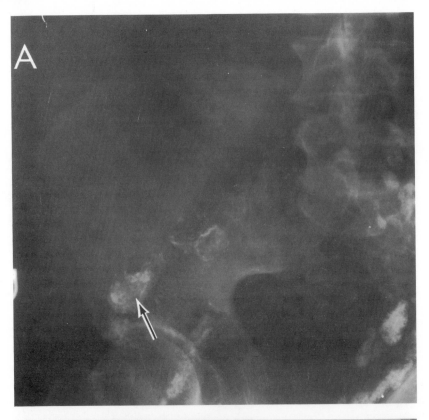

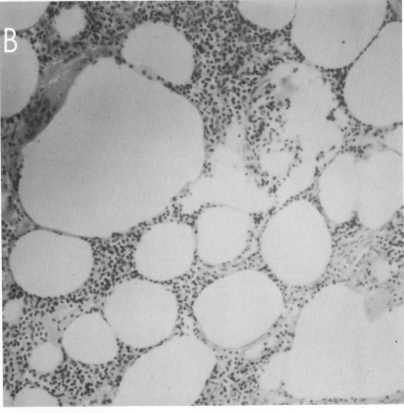

out the presence of metastatic disease and does not necessarily increase the sensitivity of testing. If histologic confirmation cannot be obtained in a study otherwise considered positive, the patient should be subjected to pelvic lymph node dissection, since false-positive errors are unacceptable.

Pelvic Lymph Node Dissection

Because of the inaccuracies of noninvasive staging of pelvic lymph nodes, pelvic lymph node dissection has been used for staging purposes in patients with apparently localized prostatic cancer. The incidence of pelvic lymph node metastases identified after surgical lymphadenectomy is dependent upon the stage and grade of the primary tumor (Table 2–2). Pelvic nodal metastasis is exceedingly rare in stage A1 tumors and has not occurred in our series.[14] On the other hand, up to one fourth of patients with stage A2 carcinoma can be expected to have positive pelvic lymph nodes detected by a node dissection. The incidence of pelvic node metastasis is around 12% in patients with stage B1 tumors, but is up to 30% in patients with stage B2 lesions. Finally, more than half the patients with extracapsular tumor extension (stage C) can be expected to have pelvic node metastasis.

Tumor grade is also a factor that influences the incidence of pelvic node metastasis. While more than half the patients with poorly differentiated tumors of any stage have pelvic node disease, only 10% of those with a well-differentiated tumor have metastasis to the pelvic lymph nodes. Overall, approximately one fourth of those with moderately differentiated tumors have pelvic lymph node metastasis.

When considered together, stage and grade of the primary tumor can be somewhat predictive of the status of the pelvic lymph nodes. The incidence of pelvic lymph node metastasis in patients with well-differentiated stage B1 tumors is less than 5%. While only 18% of patients with well-differentiated stage B2 tumors have pelvic lymph node metastasis, the incidence reaches over 40% in poorly differentiated stage B2 lesions. Finally, patients with poorly differentiated stage C tumors have more than a 90% chance of having tumor metastasis to the pelvic lymph nodes.

Despite this correlation, the stage and grade of the primary tumor cannot be used to predict accurately the status of pelvic lymph nodes in an individual patient. However, a staging error of less than 5% is probably acceptable, and most patients with well-differentiated stage B1 tumors do not require pelvic lymph node evaluation before definitive therapy. Pelvic lymph node metastasis

---

FIG 2–6.
A, filling defects and enlargement of pelvic lymph nodes interpreted as metastatic prostatic cancer. Fine-needle aspiration failed to confirm the diagnosis. **B,** after pelvic lymph node dissection, no tumor was identified but extensive fat infiltration of nodes was detected. Abnormal or suspicious lymph nodes after lymphangiography or CT scan should be confirmed histologically.

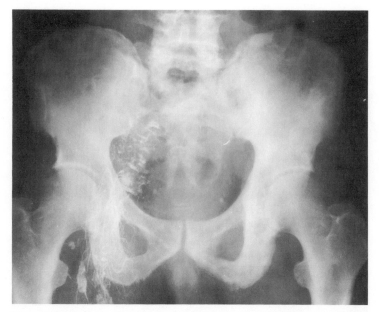

FIG 2–7.
Obstruction and replacement of right pelvic nodes by metastatic prostatic cancer.

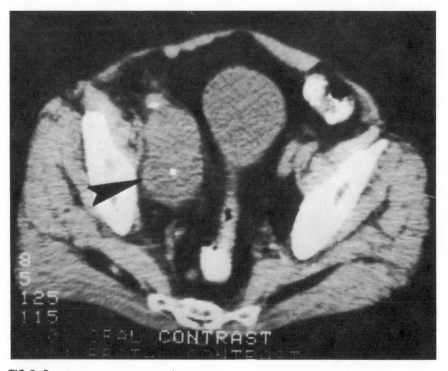

FIG 2–8.
Pelvic CT scan showing large nodal metastasis in a patient with a high-grade locally extensive tumor.

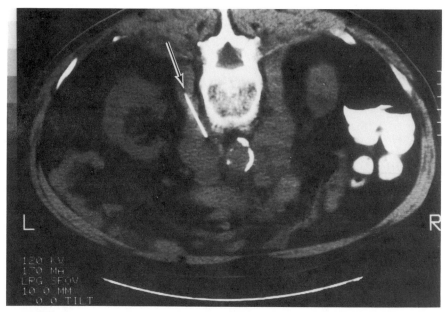

FIG 2–9.
CT-guided needle biopsy of retroperitoneal adenopathy. The tip of the needle is well visualized *(arrow)* and can be placed accurately into the abnormal area.

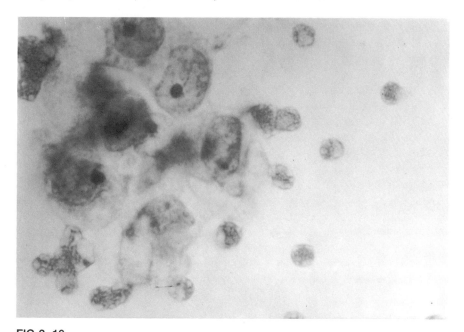

FIG 2–10.
Fine-needle aspiration from a suspicious lymph node identified on CT scan. Cells from poorly differentiated adenocarcinoma are identified. Histologic confirmation of suspicious nodes is mandatory and can eliminate false-positive staging errors.

TABLE 2–2.
Incidence of Pelvic Node Metastasis by Histologic Grade and Clinical Stage

	GRADE			
	WELL DIFFERENTIATED, NO./TOTAL (%)	MODERATELY DIFFERENTIATED, NO./TOTAL (%)	POORLY DIFFERENTIATED, NO./TOTAL (%)	TOTALS (%)
Stage				
A1	0/28	0/12	—	0/40
A2	0/7	5/19 (26)	3/8 (38)	8/34 (24)
B1	2/53 (4)	13/94 (14)	3/9 (33)	18/156 (12)
B2	5/27 (18)	29/106 (27)	9/21 (43)	43/154 (28)
C	5/10 (50)	18/44 (41)	13/14 (93)	36/68 (53)
TOTAL	**12/125** (10)	**65/275** (24)	**28/52** (54)	**105/452** (23)

in patients with stage A1 tumor is extremely rare and lymph node dissection is not indicated. In those with poorly differentiated stage C tumors nodal metastasis is exceptionally frequent. All other patients should undergo some method of lymph node evaluation prior to institution of therapy. Because of the inaccuracies of noninvasive staging techniques, most patients should undergo a surgical pelvic node dissection as a staging procedure before definitive therapy is offered.

Technique
The technique of surgical pelvic lymphadenectomy is discussed in detail in chapter 3. However, it is appropriate to review briefly the limits of a dissection performed primarily for staging purposes. The therapeutic value of lymphadenectomy is unproven, so a modified technique for pelvic lymph node dissection is used to decrease overall patient morbidity.[15]

The most commonly defined surgical obturator lymph nodes are located in a triangle subtended by the inferior border of the external iliac vein, the obturator nerve, and the endopelvic fascia. The lymph nodes lie superior to the obturator vessels and the obturator nerve. Involvement of the external iliac lymph nodes or nodes superior to the bifurcation of the common iliac artery is unusual without simultaneous metastatic disease within the anatomical boundaries described. Therefore, if a lymphadenectomy is done for staging purposes, removal of the lymphatic tissue surrounding the external iliac artery and extending over the psoas muscle to the genitofemoral nerve is unnecessary. This modification reduces operative time but, more importantly, decreases the incidence of lower extremity and genital edema. If pelvic lymphadenectomy is performed with therapeutic intent, a more extended dissection should be performed since this modified technique may underestimate the number of lymph nodes involved and does not remove all potential lymph node metastases in the pelvis. Metastases to external iliac nodes may occur as well as to a pre-sacral plexus that lies inferior and medial to the hypogastric artery.[16]

Histologic Examination

The pathologic method for examination of lymph nodes removed at the time of surgical lymphadenectomy is important. The greater the detail used in searching for metastatic deposits, the higher the incidence of pelvic lymph node metastases. Step sectioning of lymph nodes identifies metastasis in a higher percentage of patients but is not practical as a routine. In general, grossly identifiable lymph nodes are dissected from the specimen by the pathologist. They are embedded in paraffin en bloc, and representative sections of each lymph node are examined. The number of identifiable lymph nodes in the specimen varies with the extent of the dissection, the precision of the pathologist, and individual patient characteristics.

Depending upon the situation, examination of all the pelvic lymph nodes by frozen section may not be practical. In particular, this is true in a patient selected for radical retropubic prostatectomy. Frozen section evaluation of suspicious or representative lymph nodes should be performed. Most often, if the lymph nodes grossly are normal, frozen section evaluation does not detect metastatic tumor. However, the surgeon can help identify lymph nodes obtained from the primary site of potential metastasis and histologic examination by frozen section can identify microscopic tumor that otherwise was not evident. The false-negative rate is increased when frozen section examination alone of the pelvic lymph nodes is used, and around 10% of patients with grossly normal nodes and negative frozen sections are found to have microscopic metastases on permanent section examination. However, the staging error introduced by frozen section evaluation seems reasonable in this setting since wound closure and reoperation several days later after permanent sections are available is impractical.

Morbidity of Surgical Lymphadenectomy

The morbidity of surgical lymphadenectomy seems reasonable considering the information obtained by the procedure. Major vascular damage or injury to the ureter have been reported but are rare. Damage to the obturator nerve is an unusual complication. When it occurs unilaterally, the patient notices adductor weakness of the ipsilateral leg but usually suffers no significant gait abnormalities.

More common complications of lymphadenectomy are related to interruption of the lymphatic drainage of the lower extremity. With a modified dissection, significant lower-extremity or genital edema is unusual. However, a combination of whole pelvic external beam irradiation and a lymph node dissection, even by the modified technique, frequently produces lower-extremity edema. This further emphasizes the necessity for rational treatment planning before invasive procedures are performed.

Lymphocele may also occur after lymph node dissection. Careful attention should be paid to ligation or clipping of identifiable lymphatic channels, especially at the inferior portion of the dissection. The role of drains in the production or prevention of lymphoceles is uncertain, but low-dose heparin has been implicated in some patients.[17]

The most serious complication associated with pelvic lymph node dissection is pulmonary embolus. Although a concern with any operative procedure, venous thrombi may develop as a result of trauma to the external iliac vein or intraoperative retraction of the vein. Intraoperative manipulation of the external iliac vein should be kept to a minimum. Compression boots on the lower extremities may be useful, and early ambulation should be encouraged.

DETECTION OF DISTANT METASTASES

All patients with prostatic cancer in whom treatment is contemplated should undergo procedures intended to detect the presence of distant metastatic disease. As with pelvic lymph node metastasis, the presence of distant metastatic disease correlates with the stage and grade of the primary tumor. In most patients, concomitant pelvic node metastases can be identified in patients with known distant metastatic disease. Logically, studies to detect the presence of distant metastatic disease are performed prior to lymph node evaluation.

Bone

The most common site of metastatic prostate cancer beyond the pelvic lymph nodes is the bone (Fig 2–11). Presumably, tumor cells escape from the prostate via Batson's venous plexus and proceed directly to the vertebral column and skeletal system. The axial skeleton is most frequently involved. The pelvis is the most common site, followed by vertebrae, ribs, skull, and proximal extremities.[18] Some studies have suggested that the metastatic pattern of bone metastases from prostatic cancer is not unlike that seen with other tumors that frequently spread to bone, thus calling into question the significance of Batson's venous plexus.[19]

Bone Scanning

The most sensitive method for detecting bone metastases from prostatic cancer is a radionuclide bone scan. Technetium 99 methylene diphosphonate is the radiopharmaceutical agent most commonly used. Hypersensitivity reactions to this drug are extremely rare and the radioactivity to which patients are subjected is only about 1.4 rad, less than that of a chest x-ray. 2.5 mg/kg of the isotope is injected into a peripheral vein. Two hours after injection, imaging is performed. Technetium 99 accumulates in any area of increased bone turnover. Therefore, the test is not specific for prostatic cancer. However, the pattern of metastatic prostatic cancer with asymmetric uptake, frequently in the axial skeleton, is often characteristic (Fig 2–12).

Areas of degenerative arthritis may be identified but are typically symmetrical and involve the lumbar spine, the sacroiliac joints and acromio-clavicular

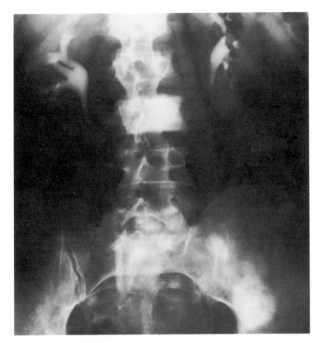

FIG 2–11.
Dense, osteoblastic lesions in L-3 vertebral body and left pelvis typical of metastatic prostate cancer.

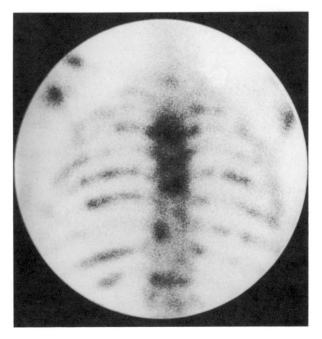

FIG 2–12.
Bone scan showing multiple areas of uptake in the ribs typical of metastatic prostatic cancer.

joints (Fig 2–13). Healing fractures also accumulate the isotope but can usually be identified as such by clinical history. Paget's disease may cause a pattern of uptake in the pelvis that is difficult to distinguish from prostatic cancer (Fig 2–14). Plain bone roentgenograms usually allow the distinction since the trabecular pattern of bone is maintained in Paget's disease (Fig 2–15). Percutaneous bone biopsy of an abnormal area identified on bone scan is rarely necessary and often yields unsatisfactory material for interpretation. Occasionally, though, the technique can be useful and gives histologic confirmation of metastatic disease in a situation that may otherwise be confusing (Fig 2–16).

Solitary lesions on bone scan may create difficulty in interpretation, but up to 10% of metastatic foci are solitary. Single abnormal areas of uptake are more likely due to cancer if they are located in the vertebrae compared to the ribs. Especially with the vertebrae and pelvis, a CT scan can be useful in determining the etiology of a solitary metastasis on bone scan since bone destruction may be evident if tumor is present (Fig 2–17).

Technetium 99 is excreted by the kidneys. Accordingly, the kidneys, bladder, and, sometimes, ureters are visualized on bone scan. Although anatomical detail is relatively imprecise, ureteral obstruction can often be detected on bone scan images. Unilateral nonvisualization of a kidney may imply longstanding obstruction or some other insult that has resulted in nonfunction. Bilateral nonvisualization of the kidneys should raise the question of a "superscan" (Fig 2–18). When widespread diffuse metastatic disease is present, bone deposition

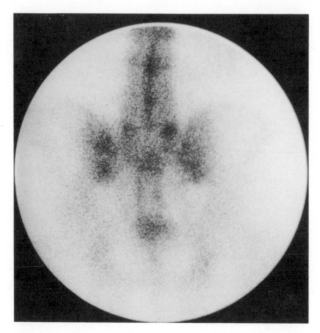

FIG 2–13.
Abnormal bone scan from degenerative joint disease. The characteristic location is helpful in distinguishing degenerative disease from metastatic cancer.

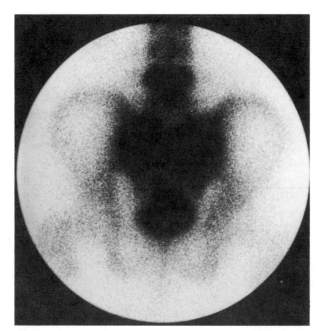

FIG 2–14.
Bone scan showing intense uptake from Paget's disease. The symmetry as well as the characteristic location is helpful in distinguishing Paget's disease from metastatic prostatic cancer.

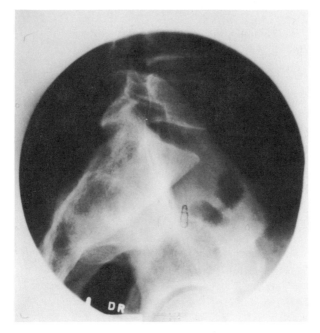

FIG 2–15.
Lateral view of pelvis and sacrum showing typical changes of Paget's disease. The trabecular pattern of bone is maintained or increased in Paget's disease.

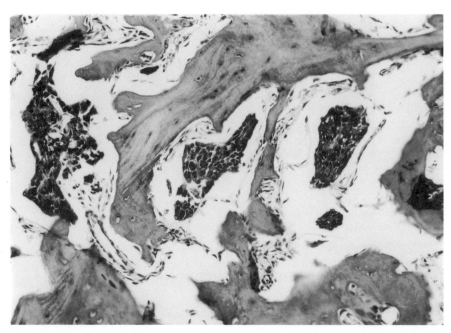

FIG 2–16.
Bone biopsy showing metastatic adenocarcinoma. Bone biopsy rarely is necessary to confirm the diagnosis but occasionally is useful in patients with equivocal bone scans.

of the radiopharmaceutical may decrease circulating levels of the agent such that renal excretion and visualization are minimized. If the uptake is diffuse and symmetrical, the gain may be decreased before printing of the scan and a false-negative interpretation may result. The absence of renal excretion of the radiopharmaceutical agent and minimal soft-tissue visualization are the keys to avoidance of false-negative interpretation of a superscan.[20]

Bone Roentgenograms

Most bone metastases from prostatic cancer are blastic in nature and often can be visualized on plain bone roentgenograms (Fig 2–19). Increased bone density with loss of the trabecular pattern is seen. However, bone roentgenograms are relatively insensitive since a substantial percentage of the bone must be replaced by tumor before lesions are visible. Tumor cells produce bone destruction, but a reactive hyperplasia of the bone occurs resulting in a typical osteoblastic lesion. Not all metastases from prostatic cancer are osteoblastic. Osteolytic alone and mixed osteoblastic and osteolytic lesions may also be seen, even in the same patient.

Other conditions may produce changes on skeletal roentgenograms that are similar to those seen with prostatic cancer. Rests of dense cortical bone known as bone islands may mimic metastases from prostatic cancer. Degenerative bone changes usually can be distinguished from prostatic cancer by their symmetry and typical location. Paget's disease produces a pattern that may be difficult to distinguish from prostatic cancer on bone scan and can also create confusion on bone roentgenograms. Typically, bone trabeculation is maintained or even increased in patients with Paget's disease, whereas the trabecular pattern often is obscured in patients with prostatic cancer. Paget's disease frequently involves the pelvis and sacroiliac region and may have a more symmetric uptake than prostatic cancer.

Skeletal roentgenograms are less sensitive than radionuclide bone scans.[21] However, films of appropriate areas identified on bone scan may be useful in increasing the specificity of staging. Also, bone roentgenograms of lesions in the humerus or femur identified on bone scan should be obtained to rule out impending pathologic fracture.

Soft-Tissue Metastases

Soft-tissue metastases from prostatic cancer usually are recognized at autopsy or in end-stage patients. However, soft-tissue disease may occur in the absence of demonstrable bone metastases. Metastases from prostatic cancer can occur in virtually any area of the body.

A chest x-ray should be obtained as a staging procedure in all patients

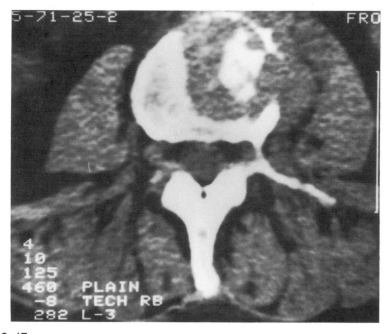

FIG 2–17.
CT scan showing destruction of left side of vertebral body with soft-tissue mass from metastatic carcinoma of the prostate. CT scans may be particularly useful in determining the nature of abnormal uptake in the spine on a bone scan.

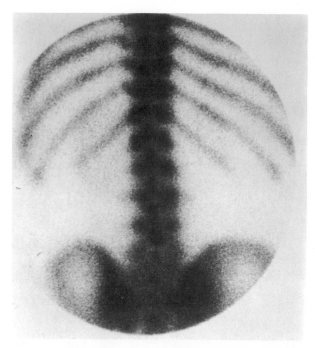

FIG 2–18.
Portion of a superscan in a patient with widespread metastases from prostatic cancer. The lack of renal excretion as well as the absence of background soft-tissue uptake are typical.

with prostatic cancer. Metastatic deposits of prostatic cancer may form typical round lesions within the lung but often present as an interstitial infiltrative process (Fig 2–20). Blastic lesions in the ribs may also be detected.

Liver metastasis is generally an ominous prognostic sign in patients with prostatic cancer (Fig 2–21). However, the infrequency with which this occurs makes liver scanning or CT scans of the liver unnecessary on a routine basis. Proptosis due to retro-orbital metastases has been reported but, in general, brain metastases are unusual.

Physical examination occasionally reveals evidence of metastatic prostatic cancer. Palpable adenopathy may occur in the supraclavicular region or in the inguinal lymph nodes. Metastasis to the corpora cavernosa is seen in some patients, and metastatic involvement of the testis or epididymis has been reported.

CHEMICAL AND ENZYMATIC MARKERS

Routine serum chemistry studies should be obtained in all patients with prostatic cancer. Elevation of serum BUN or creatinine levels may indicate the presence of ureteral obstruction. Abnormal liver function test results can lead to appropriate studies to detect liver metastasis. In addition, serum hemoglobin values should be obtained. Anemia of chronic disease may occur, but profound suppression of hemoglobin levels may also be seen in patients with widespread metastases and replacement of bone marrow by tumor cells. Overall, though, the most useful blood studies in the staging of prostatic cancer are serum acid and alkaline phosphatase as well as prostate specific antigen.

Acid Phosphatase

Traditionally, the most specific and sensitive biochemical marker for prostatic cancer has been serum acid phosphatase. In general, elevation of serum acid phosphatase levels implies extracapsular tumor extension, although some of the more sensitive assays reportedly can detect intracapsular tumor in some patients. The mechanism behind the elevation of serum acid phosphatase in prostatic cancer patients is uncertain. The acid phosphatase content of prostatic adenocarcinoma cells is less than that of the normal prostate or the cells of benign prostatic hyperplasia. Under normal conditions, acid phosphatase is

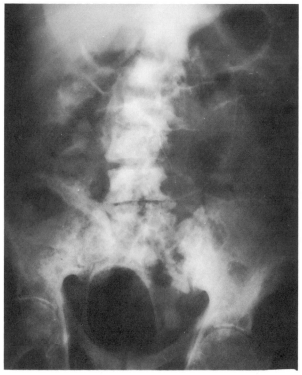

FIG 2–19.
Typical blastic changes in bone due to metastatic prostatic cancer.

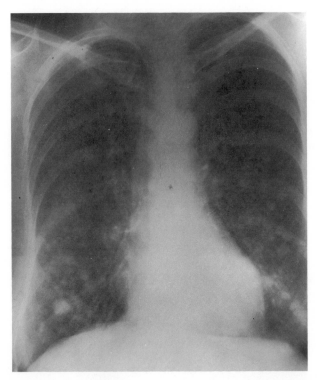

FIG 2–20.
Chest x-ray showing diffuse interstitial infiltrates from metastatic prostatic cancer. Lung metastases from prostatic cancer often result in a diffuse infiltrative pattern rather than nodular metastases.

secreted by the acinar cells and released into the seminal fluid. Levels of acid phosphatase in prostatic fluid are markedly higher than those found in the serum. Presumably, acid phosphatase is released into the serum in patients with prostatic cancer because the normal conduction system for release of acid phosphatase into the seminal fluid is altered by the neoplastic process.

Early methods for measurement of serum acid phosphatase by colorimetric determination led to false-positive results because of the inability to distinguish between acid phosphatase of prostatic origin and that produced by other tissues. Acid phosphatases are a heterogeneous group of isoenzymes, and elevated serum levels may be observed in patients with pancreatic cancer, osteosarcoma, thrombocytopenia, thromboembolic diseases, leukemia, and polycythemia vera.[22] Acid phosphatases produced in the prostate are not measurable in normal serum. However, some of the same isoenzymes are contained within neutrophils and may be detected in the serum of patients with abnormalities of neutrophils such as granulocytic leukemia. Various techniques for determination of serum acid phosphatase have been developed. The sensitivity and specificity depends upon the method used.

Enzymatic Methods

Most often, enzymatic methods are used for determination of serum acid phosphatase levels. Most laboratories report a total acid phosphatase level as well as a prostatic specific acid phosphatase value. When enzymatic methods are used, false-positive elevations of serum acid phosphatase are uncommon. A reproducible elevation of acid phosphatase usually implies the presence of extracapsular tumor. On the other hand, enzymatic determination of serum acid phosphatase is relatively insensitive, and as many as 20% or 30% of patients with demonstrable metastatic disease may have normal levels.

Radioimmunoassay

Radioimmunoassay (RIA) has been found to be a more sensitive but less specific method for determination of serum acid phosphatase levels. Initially, it was believed that this test could detect intracapsular disease in a significant number of patients. Therefore, it was proposed as a method for screening wide segments of the population.[23] However, the incidence of false-positive results makes it impractical as a screening method. Also, the lack of specificity and the false-positive rates introduce potential confusion in interpretation of results in patients with otherwise localized disease. Overall, RIA determination of prostatic acid phosphatase levels has proven to be no more useful than

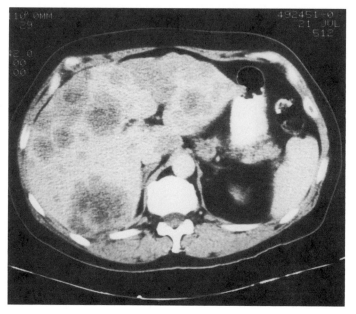

FIG 2–21.
CT scan showing metastatic tumor in the liver. Clinically evident liver metastasis usually is seen only in patients with widespread tumor, especially in bones.

specific enzymatic methods either as an initial staging procedure in patients with prostatic cancer or for following treatment response.[24]

Counterimmunoelectrophoresis

Counterimmunoelectrophoresis (CIEP) is another technique for acid phosphatase determination that initially was thought to have a sensitivity that could increase its overall usefulness for staging prostatic cancer.[25] In addition, CIEP has been mentioned as a potential screening test for prostatic cancer. Like RIA, false-positive rates with CIEP negate its usefulness as a screening test and introduce possible sources for error in making clinical decisions based upon acid phosphatase levels alone.

Bone Marrow Acid Phosphatase

Acid phosphatase determinations on bone marrow aspirates have also been used in an attempt to increase the sensitivity of the test. Enzymatic methods generally have been unsuitable for bone marrow aspirates. Schellhammer et al.[26] found elevated serum levels of acid phosphatase in nearly 95% of patients having abnormal bone marrow acid measured by CIEP. Similarly, RIA acid phosphatase determinations on bone marrow aspirates have yielded little information not obtainable from serum levels.[27]

Clinical Interpretation of Acid Phosphatase Results

Although acid phosphatase can be a useful marker for following the response to therapy in patients with prostatic cancer, the interpretation of results in a specific patient can be confusing. Presumably, acid phosphatase levels can be elevated in some patients with intracapsular disease, especially when determinations are made by RIA or CIEP. However, it has been demonstrated that patients with elevated serum acid phosphatase levels have a poor long-term prognosis even in the presence of histologically negative lymph nodes and tumors that palpably are confined within the prostatic capsule.[28] Despite this, we have not excluded patients from definitive treatment based upon modest elevation of acid phosphatase alone.

Abnormal acid phosphatase levels should be confirmed by repeated determination. Variation in serum levels, either on a circadian pattern[28] or at random,[29] have been demonstrated. Also, prostatic manipulation either by rectal examination or cystoscopy can cause false-positive elevations of serum acid phosphatase levels if the blood sample is drawn within a few days of the manipulation. While this does not necessarily imply that blood samples should not be drawn after rectal examination, it does indicate that a repeated sample should be obtained several days later if the initial levels are found to be elevated.

The degree of elevation of serum acid phosphatase may correlate with prognosis although this may simply be a reflection of tumor bulk. The data from the Veterans Administration Cooperative Urologic Group indicated that serum acid phosphatase levels at the upper limit of normal but within the normal range implied a worse prognosis than levels at the lower limit of normal.[30] However, once the acid phosphatase concentration is elevated, the correlation between the absolute value and prognosis is inexact. Indeed, some tumors do not produce acid phosphatase despite large tumor burden.

Alkaline Phosphatase

Alkaline phosphatase levels often are elevated in patients with bone metastases from prostatic cancer. Presumably, increased bone metabolism surrounding the osseous metastases accounts for the elevation. Alkaline phosphatase is less specific than acid phosphatase as a marker for prostatic cancer. In addition, a phenomenon of alkaline phosphatase flare may be seen after the institution of endocrine therapy wherein acute elevations or further increases in the serum alkaline phosphatase level are observed due to healing bone metastases. Alkaline phosphatase is elevated in any situation in which increased bone metabolism is present, including Paget's disease. Alkaline phosphatase of hepatic origin can be distinguished from that produced by bone since that from the liver is heat stable while alkaline phosphatase of bone origin is heat labile.

Prostate-Specific Antigen

A human prostate-specific antigen (PSA) was reported in 1979 and appears to be more sensitive for prostatic cancer than prostatic acid phosphatase.[31] Although PSA levels may be elevated even when disease is localized, the trend is toward higher levels with more advanced stages.[32] It seems unlikely that PSA will be useful for screening of the general population. However, it has been shown to be a very sensitive and specific marker for disease progression following hormonal therapy or for detection of recurrent disease after radical prostatectomy. In addition, it is of use in the differential diagnosis of metastatic carcinomas of unknown primary or in distinguishing poorly differentiated prostatic cancer invading the bladder neck or trigone from transitional cell carcinoma.[33] Prostate-specific antigen likely will play an increasing role in the clinical management of prostatic cancer as more data regarding its sensitivities and variabilities emerge.

REFERENCES

1. Jewett HJ: The present status of radical prostatectomy for stages A and B prostatic cancer. *Urol Clin North Am* 1975; 2:105–124.
2. Bartsch G, Dietze O, Hohlbrugger G, et al: Incidental carcinoma of the prostate—grading and tumor volume in relation to survival rate. *World J Urol* 1983; 1:24–28.

3. Guinan P, Bush I, Ray V, et al: The accuracy of the rectal examination in the diagnosis of prostate carcinoma. *N Engl J Med* 1980; 303:499.

4. Elder JS, Jewett HJ, Walsh PC: Radical perineal prostatectomy for clinical stage B2 carcinoma of the prostate. *J Urol* 1982; 127:704–706.

5. Smith JA Jr, Middleton RG: Radical prostatectomy for stage B2 carcinoma of the prostate. *J Urol* 1982; 127:702–703.

6. Resnick MI: Ultrasonography in the detection and diagnosis of carcinoma of the prostate. *Cancer Detec Prevent* 1979; 2:625.

7. Lee F, McLeary R, Kumsaka G: Prostate cancer: Diagnosis by transrectal ultrasound. *J Urol* 1986; 135:147A.

8. Cohen JM, Resnick MI: The use of transrectal ultrasonography in the diagnosis of stage A prostatic carcinoma. *World J Urol* 1983; 1:12–14.

9. Scardino PT, Wheeler TM, Shinohara K, et al: Confined or not confined: The value of transrectal ultrasonography in staging prostatic cancer. *J Urol* 1986; 135:149A.

10. Merrin C, Wajsman Z, Baumgartner G, et al: The clinical value of lymphangiography: Are the nodes surrounding the obturator nerve visualized? *J Urol* 1977; 117:762–764.

11. Correa RJ Jr, Kidd CR, Burnett L, et al: Percutaneous pelvic lymph node aspiration in carcinoma of the prostate. *J Urol* 1981; 126:190–191.

12. Weinerman PM, Arger PH, Coleman BG, et al: Pelvic and bladder adenopathy from bladder and prostate carcinoma: Detection by rapid sequence computer tomography. *Am J Radiol* 1983; 140:95–99.

13. Wajsman Z, Gamarra M, Park JJ, et al: Transabdominal fine-needle aspiration of retroperitoneal lymph nodes in staging of genitourinary tract cancer: Correlation with lymphography and lymph node dissection findings. *J Urol* 1982; 128:1238–1240.

14. Smith JA Jr, Seaman JP, Gleidman JB, et al: Pelvic lymph node metastasis from prostatic cancer: Influence of tumor grade and stage in 452 consecutive patients. *J Urol* 1983; 130:290–292.

15. Fisher H, Herr H, Sogani P, et al: Modified pelvic lymph node dissection in patients undergoing I-125 implantation for carcinoma of the prostate, presented at the American Urological Association meeting, 1981, abstract No. 299.

16. Golimbu M, Morales P, Al-Askari S, et al: Extended pelvic lymphadenectomy for prostatic cancer. *J Urol* 1979; 121:617–620.

17. Sogani PC, Watson RC, Whitmore WF Jr: Lymphocele after pelvic lymphadenectomy for urologic cancer. *Urology* 1981; 17:39–43.

18. Tafe AJ, Francis MD, Harvey WJ: Correlation of neoplasms with incidence and localization of skeletal metastases: An analysis of 1,355 diphosphonate bone scans. *J Nucl Med* 1975; 16:986–989.

19. Robey EL, Schellhammer PF: Solitary lesions on bone scan in genitourinary malignancy. *J Urol* 1984; 132:1002.

20. Constable AR, Cranage RW: Recognition of the superscan in prostate bone scintigraphy. *Br J Radiol* 1981; 54:112–125.

21. McNeil BJ: Value of bone scanning in neoplastic disease. *Semin Nucl Med* 1984; 14:277–286.

22. Heneberry MO, Engel G, Grayhack JT: Acid phosphatase. *Urol Clin North Am* 1979; 6:629–641.

23. Foti AG, Cooper JF, Herschman H, et al: Detection of prostatic cancer by solid-

phase radioimmunoassay of serum prostatic acid phosphatase. *N Engl J Med* 1977; 297:1357–1361.

24. Pontes JE, Choe BK, Rose NR, et al: Clinical evaluation of immunologic methods for detection of serum prostatic acid phosphatase. *J Urol* 1981; 126:363–365.

25. Chu TM, Wang MC, Scott WW, et al: Immunochemical detection of serum prostatic acid phosphatase: Methodology and clinical evaluation. *Invest Urol* 1978; 15:319–323.

26. Schellhammer PF, Warden SS, Wright GL, et al: Boen marrow acid phosphatase by counterimmune electrophoresis: Pretreatment and post-treatment correlations. *J Urol* 1982; 127:66–68.

27. Pontes JE, Choe B, Rose N, et al: Reliability of bone marrow acid phosphatase as a parameter of metastatic prostatic cancer. *J Urol* 1979; 122:178–179.

28. Doe RP, Mellinger GT: Circadian variation of serum acid phosphatase in prostatic cancer. *Metabolism* 1964; 13:445–452.

29. Nissenkorn I, Mickey DD, Miller DB, et al: Circadian and day-to-day variation of prostatic acid phosphatase. *J Urol* 1982; 127:1122–1124.

30. Byar DP, Corle DK: Veterans Administration Cooperative Urologic Research Group: VACURG randomization trial of radical prostatectomy for stages I and II prostate cancer. *Urology* 1983; 17:7–11.

31. Want MC, Valenzuala LA, Murphy GP, et al: Purification of a human prostate specific antigen. *Invest Urol* 1979; 17:159–163.

32. Ming Chu T, Murphy GP: What's new in tumor markers for prostatic cancer? *Urology* 1986; 27:487–491.

33. Lange PH, Ercole CJ, Vesselle RL: Tumor markers in the follow-up of initial therapy of prostatic cancer, in Lange PH (ed): *Tumor Markers in Prostatic Cancer.* Princeton, NJ, Excerpta Medica, 1986, pp 16–23.

3

Methods of Definitive Local Therapy

There are, perhaps, fewer areas in medicine that generate more disagreement than the appropriate management of localized prostatic cancer. To a great extent, the confusion surrounding this subject is due to the variable natural history of the disease and its occurrence in a patient population that generally is of an advanced age and with many competing causes of death. Very few randomized studies have been conducted comparing the various forms of treatment for localized prostatic cancer. Comparisons between retrospective series often are invalid because of variability in patient selection and staging. Therefore, there are no definitive data that allow the clinician to make dogmatic recommendations regarding selection of therapy. Nevertheless, the concept that the patient will "make the choice" is not truly feasible and, to some degree, is unfair to patients. Although patient wishes clearly should be paramount in deciding upon selection of definitive therapy or even the need to proceed with such treatment, it is incumbent upon the clinician to make well-informed recommendations that are in concert with the specifics of an individual patient's situation.

It is not the purpose of this chapter to discuss the advantages and disadvantages of various forms of treatment for localized prostatic cancer. Treatment options and the rationale for certain recommendations are discussed in detail in the various chapters dealing with the specific stages of prostatic cancer. Rather, this chapter discusses the technique, complications, and side effects of various treatment methods. Selection of therapy and appropriate applications for specific stages of the disease are discussed elsewhere.

RADICAL PROSTATECTOMY

Radical prostatectomy implies surgical removal of the entire prostate gland and prostatic capsule as well as the seminal vesicles. In selected patients, good long-term (greater than 15 years) disease-free survival rates have been demonstrated after radical prostatectomy. Appropriately, it is sometimes argued that patients who have a favorable result from radical prostatectomy often are the same ones who likely have a relatively indolent and slowly progressive tumor. At any rate, the role of radical prostatectomy as curative therapy for some prostatic cancers is well established. Recent technical innovations that have decreased the overall morbidity of the procedure have increased interest in the operation and have led to more frequent application of the procedure.

Patient Selection

Patients with tumor that apparently is confined within the capsule of the prostate gland are candidates for radical prostatectomy. This includes patients with stage A and stage B prostatic cancer. Since the margin of surgical dissection in radical prostatectomy follows closely along the prostatic capsule, it seems logical that surgical margins are inadequate in patients with extracapsular extension of tumor. Therefore, the procedure does not seem indicated in patients with obvious tumor extension beyond the capsule of the prostate.

In general, patients should have a reasonable expectancy of 10 to 15 years of life in order to justify the operation. Many years may elapse before stage A or stage B prostatic cancer becomes clinically significant even in the absence of therapeutic intervention, so radical prostatectomy should be reserved for patients in whom the tumor is likely to represent a threat to health. Usually, this includes patients younger than 75 years who are otherwise in relatively good condition. Obviously, however, any age limit for the operation is entirely arbitrary, and chronological age alone is only one criterion that should be considered.

Some authors have recommended radical prostatectomy for stage C prostatic cancer and have achieved apparently good results.[2,3] In most series, adjuvant therapy (usually hormonal treatment) has been used. The operation has also been performed in some patients with stage C prostatic cancer as palliation or prevention of local symptoms. Local symptoms from prostatic cancer usually can be managed adequately by other means, and radical prostatectomy is not justified in most patients simply for palliation of potential local problems.

Since radical prostatectomy is a form of local therapy, patients with histologic evidence of lymph node metastasis should be excluded. Lymphadenectomy usually is considered to be a staging procedure alone with little therapeutic value. As discussed in chapter 7, radical prostatectomy with early hormonal therapy has been performed in some patients with proven pelvic lymph node metastases, but long-term disease-free survival rates are not known.[4]

Patient Preparation

Staging procedures including chest x-ray films, serum acid phosphatase evaluations, and bone scanning are performed prior to the decision to proceed with radical prostatectomy. In addition, careful digital palpation of the prostate should show no evidence of extraprostatic induration or extension into the seminal vesicles. If CT scanning or other imaging of the prostate has not been completed, an IV pyelogram should be performed to rule out ureteral obstruction. Often, the visualization of the kidneys and ureters on a bone scan is sufficient and pyelography is not necessary.

Any urine infection should have been cleared preoperatively by antibiotics. If the patient is in urinary retention and has an indwelling Foley catheter, perioperative antibiotics should be administered. Otherwise, the routine use of antibiotics in the perioperative period is not necessary. Preoperative anticoagulation with low-dose heparin is not used since this has been shown to increase bleeding complications and, possibly, lymphocele formation.[5]

Rectal injury is an unusual but possible complication of radical prostatectomy. Therefore, a complete mechanical and antibiotic preparation of the bowel may be used. In general, though, this seems unnecessary and cleansing enemas the night prior to surgery usually suffice.

SURGICAL TECHNIQUE

Pelvic Lymphadenectomy

Lymph node dissection is performed as a staging procedure prior to radical prostatectomy. Accordingly, the operation should be limited in scope, but the surgical dissection should encompass the primary lymphatic drainage of the prostate. Description of lymph node groups in the pelvis is largely a matter of semantics, but the operation is designed to remove the obturator and hypogastric lymph nodes as well as nodes along the medial external iliac chain (Fig 3–1).

The procedure can be performed under general, spinal, or epidural anesthesia, but sufficient abdominal relaxation is necessary. Patients are placed in the supine position. A Foley catheter should be passed through the urethra to decompress the bladder and facilitate its retraction from the operative field. Often, it is useful to flex the table and place the patient in a slight Trendelenburg position in order to lift the pelvis into the field and allow gravity to help displace the peritoneal contents. A midline incision is made from just below the umbilicus to the pubis. Alternatively, bilateral sequential lower-quadrant incisions have been described when lymphadenectomy is performed as an independent procedure.[6] Extraperitoneal exposure of the lateral pelvic wall is obtained by blunt dissection of the peritoneal envelope medially and superiorly. The dissection plane is just below the epigastric vessels. Division of the vas deferens may facilitate superior retraction of the peritoneum. A self-retaining retractor such as a Balfour is placed for added exposure.

The anatomical limits of the dissection are the midpoint of the external iliac artery laterally and a point approximately 1 cm proximal to the bifurcation of the common iliac artery superiorly. Inferiorly, the dissection extends to the level of the node of Cloquet, a point identified by the circumflex iliac vein that

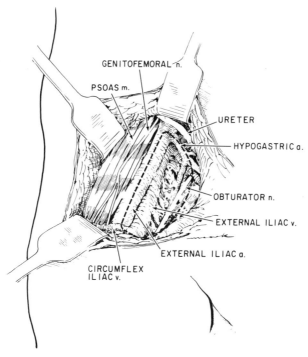

FIG 3–1.
Pelvic anatomy for modified pelvic lymph node dissection as a staging procedure for carcinoma of the prostate. The dotted line highlights the area of the dissection.

crosses the external iliac artery. The medial margin of dissection is the bladder, and the lymphadenectomy extends posteriorly to the obturator nerve. It is not routinely necessary to sacrifice the obturator vessels that lie posterior to the nerve. Generally, there is minimal lymphatic tissue posterior to the nerve, and large venous ramifications of the internal iliac system can cause troublesome bleeding in this area. However, dissection should be complete along the hypogastric artery near the bifurcation of the common iliac artery. The ureter should be identified in this area and retracted medially and superiorly. Hemoclips should be used liberally on lymphatic vessels, especially at the inferior and superior margins.

Once the dissection has been completed, the specimen is sent for frozen-section examination. Any suspicious lymph nodes should be marked appropriately and specific examination of these areas requested. If the lymph nodes grossly appear normal, the contralateral dissection can be completed in the same manner while frozen-section analysis of the first side is being completed. If there is gross nodal disease or a frozen section that confirms metastatic tumor, there is no need to proceed with contralateral lymphadenectomy, since the procedure is considered to be useful for staging purposes only and generally is not performed for therapeutic reasons.

Based on the premise that tumor spread will likely occur to ipsilateral lymph nodes, a unilateral dissection alone has been mentioned as a way to decrease morbidity. While there is a tendency for ipsilateral metastatic spread and we initiate the dissection on the side of the palpable tumor nodule, cross-over to contralateral lymphatics has occurred in the absence of identifiable ipsilateral metastasis. Furthermore, once the unilateral dissection has been completed, the morbidity of performing a contralateral limited node dissection as described is negligible. Therefore, there is little reason or incentive for performing a unilateral dissection unless nodal metastases are identified.

Once lymphadenectomy is completed, radical retropubic prostatectomy commences if the results of frozen-section examination are normal. If the procedure is performed as a separate staging maneuver or prior to radical perineal prostatectomy, the incision is closed. Penrose drains are not used if lymphadenectomy alone is performed.

Complications

The complications of pelvic lymphadenectomy alone can be assessed from series in which the operation was performed as a separate staging procedure, usually before a planned radical perineal prostatectomy. Most of the patients in these series underwent extended lymphadenectomy rather than the more limited, modified dissection more commonly performed now.[7]

Pelvic lymphadenectomy is associated with the complications inherent to any surgical procedure including pneumonia, wound infection, and a low incidence of postoperative problems such as myocardial infarction and cerebral vascular accidents. Several potential complications deserve special comment, however. First of all, postoperative lymphocele may develop, usually manifested by pelvic pain or lower-extremity edema.[8] Bladder displacement may be seen on cystogram. If the lymphocele is relatively small and symptoms are minimal, expectant therapy is appropriate since gradual resolution can be anticipated. Otherwise, percutaneous aspiration may be sufficient, although occasionally open drainage of the lymphocele is necessary. Marsupialization of the lymphocele to the peritoneum is rarely necessary. Lymphocele formation appears to be somewhat increased in patients treated with low-dose heparin preoperatively.[5] Meticulous use of hemoclips on identifiable lymphatic vessels during surgery, particularly at the proximal and distal limits of the dissection, can help decrease the incidence of postoperative lymphocele formation.

Lower-extremity and genital edema due to interruption of lymphatic drainage from the leg have been seen in some patients undergoing extended lymphadenectomy. This is unusual after a more limited, modified dissection that preserves the lymphatic channels surrounding the external iliac artery and those between the artery and the genitofemoral nerve. When pelvic irradiation is used, even after a limited dissection, edema may develop from fibrosis of other lymphatic channels within the pelvis.

Intraoperative injury to the external iliac artery or vein can occur but usually is repairable using fine monofilament suture. Typically, there are no branches of the external iliac artery within the pelvis. In some patients, though, posterior branches of the external iliac vein are identified. An accessory obturator vein not infrequently arises from the external iliac vein and the circumflex iliac vein is a relatively constant finding. Identification of these branches helps prevent injury, but routine ligation and division is not necessary. Intraoperative injury to the obturator nerve may also occur. The functional morbidity associated with unilateral division of the obturator nerve usually is relatively minimal. The patient notices some adductor weakness, but ambulation is relatively normal. If the nerve is severed, reapproximation of the ends using fine monofilament suture may allow some functional return. Damage to the ureter has been reported but should be easily avoidable by identification and medial retraction.

Deep venous thrombosis or pulmonary embolus has been reported to occur in approximately 2% of patients. Care should be taken during surgery to avoid excessive manipulation and retraction of the external iliac vein. Intraoperative leg wraps or intermittent compression boots as well as early postoperative ambulation may also be useful.

Radical Prostatectomy

Radical prostatectomy implies complete removal of the prostate and prostatic capsule as well as the seminal vesicles. Little surrounding soft tissue is removed along with the specimen, and the margin of resection relatively closely approximates the prostatic capsule. Radical prostatectomy was the first form of definitive treatment used for prostatic cancer. The procedure was popularized by Young in 1905, who used the perineal route.[10] In 1948, radical retropubic prostatectomy was described by Millen.[11] The surgical specimen is similar with both approaches, and neither has been shown to have any therapeutic advantage over the other. The choice of prostatectomy depends to some extent upon the preference and experience of the individual surgeon. Recent refinements in surgical technique allow preservation of potency in some patients undergoing radical retropubic prostatectomy.[12] Also, a staging pelvic lymphadenectomy can be performed simultaneously and through the same incision as a radical retropubic prostatectomy. When pelvic lymphadenectomy is not necessary and erectile potency is not an issue, the perineal approach becomes more attractive.

Radical Perineal Prostatectomy

The radical perineal approach for prostatectomy has been used less frequently recently because, when associated with pelvic lymph node dissection, the procedure requires two incisions. Radical perineal prostatectomy can be performed under the same anesthetic as for the pelvic node dissection and frozen-section evaluation. Alternatively, staged procedures can be utilized, with radical prostatectomy being performed after permanent sections of the lymph nodes are available. More recently, patients have been selected for radical per-

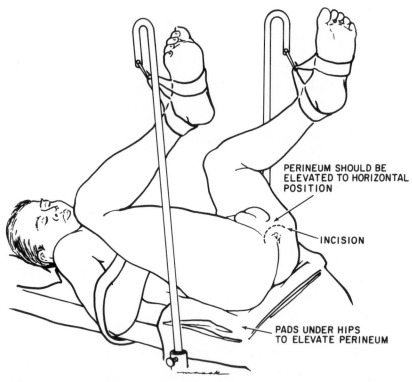

FIG 3–2.
Patient positioning for radical perineal prostatectomy. An exaggerated lithotomy position is used with the perineum elevated to a horizontal position.

ineal prostatectomy if the stage of their primary tumor is such that the incidence of pelvic lymph node metastasis is extremely low (i.e., well-differentiated clinical stage B1 tumors).[13]

Patients are placed in an exaggerated lithotomy position (Fig 3–2). Sandbags or folded towels are used to elevate the perineum to the horizontal position. An inverted "U" incision is made with the apex of the incision several centimeters anterior to the anal verge. As the incision is carried through the subcutaneous tissue, the ischiorectal fossa can be developed bluntly at each lateral margin of the incision. At this point, the central tendon is identified. The central tendon is a confluence of muscle fibers and fascia that connects to the perineal body. These fibers should be incised sharply. The levator ani muscles are retracted laterally and the bulbospongiosus muscle is retracted anteriorly.

After this, the rectourethralis muscle is encountered. It is at this point in the operation that the greatest risk of rectal injury exists. The rectum is lifted anteriorly by the rectourethralis muscle. The muscle itself must be divided close to the prostate. After this, the rectum falls away from the prostate and can be retracted posteriorly. A Lowsley retractor facilitates this dissection. The Lowsley is passed into the bladder and the blades opened. Anterior pressure on the Lowsley allows presentation of the prostate into the operative field.

An alternative approach to the prostate is to proceed in a plane posterior to the muscles of the anal sphincter. This approach, described by Belt and colleagues,[14] is a modification of the original operation of Young. It allows early identification of the rectum and dissection along the plane of the rectum posterior to the anal sphincter. The sphincter can be retracted anteriorly. If appropriate caution is used in dividing the rectourethralis muscle, this approach becomes unnecessary and the overall exposure seems slightly less optimal than that obtained through the suprasphincteric approach.

After the rectourethralis muscle is divided, Denonvilliers' fascia should be visible. This is a distinct, white fascial layer descriptively called the "pearly gates." An incision is made in the posterior layer of Denonvilliers' fascia. Using the blunt end of a knife, the fascia can then be stripped from the posterior capsule of the prostate. Further posteriorly, the ampullae of the vasa deferentia and the base of the seminal vesicles are visualized (Fig 3–3).

After the posterior surface of the prostate has been mobilized well by blunt dissection, the prostatic apex and urethra can clearly be identified. A curved clamp is passed around the membranous urethra and the urethra is

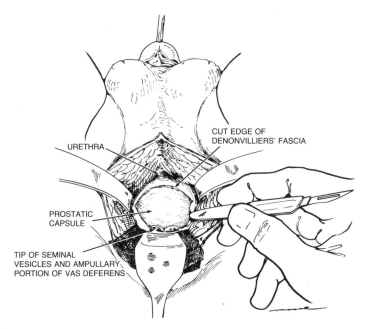

FIG 3–3.
Exposure of the prostate by the perineal route. The rectum is retracted inferiorly and the seminal vesicles and vasa deferentia are visualized.

divided just at the apex of the prostate. Bleeding from the dorsal vein complex, a frequent problem during the radical retropubic approach, generally is not encountered during radical perineal prostatectomy. The plane of dissection usually lies posterior to the dorsal vein complex. The Lowsley retractor is removed and a Young prostatic tractor is passed through the prostate and into the bladder. This allows exposure of the bladder neck, and an incision into the bladder is made just above the anterior border of the prostate. Five milliliters of indigo carmine should be given intravenously to facilitate identification of the ureteral orifices later. The prostate is separated from the bladder neck by sharp dissection. Small bleeders are cauterized as they are encountered, but clamping and ligatures may be required for some vessels.

As the bladder base and trigone are approached, care should be taken to identify the ureteral orifices. The indigo carmine injected earlier facilitates identification. Ureteral catheters may be inserted at this point but are not mandatory if the orifices are well visualized. An incision is made in the bladder trigone distal to the ureteral orifices.

The remainder of the prostatic pedicle entering posterolaterally is identified and the vessels are ligated with absorbable suture. The bladder base is elevated from the tip of the seminal vesicles, which can be dissected free in their entirety. The artery at the tip of the seminal vesicles should be clipped or tied. The vasa deferentia are also ligated and divided. The entire specimen—consisting of the prostate and prostatic capsule as well as the seminal vesicles and ampullary portion of the vasa deferentia—is then removed.

After hemostasis is obtained, the bladder neck is closed in a racket handle fashion extending from posterior to anterior.[15] Interrupted sutures of 2–0 chromic are used for closure (Fig 3–4). Care should be taken to avoid incorporating the ureteral orifices or ureters in the closing sutures. Visualization for vesicourethral anastomosis is usually excellent and superior to that obtained by the retropubic approach. A 20 French Foley catheter is passed through the urethra, and interrupted 2–0 chromic sutures are used to approximate the anterior portion of the racket handle closure to the membranous urethra. Mucosa should be included in the anastomotic sutures, but incorporation of the muscles and other tissues that surround the membranous urethra is neither necessary nor desirable. After the anastomosis is complete, the catheter is irrigated to make certain that the anastomosis is relatively watertight. Two small Penrose drains are brought out through the lateral portions of the incision. The incision is then closed with a 3–0 absorbable suture and the central tendon area is reapproximated.

Postoperatively, early ambulation is encouraged. The incision should be painted with betadine, and a heat lamp can be used to help dry the tissue and prevent maceration. The Penrose drain is left indwelling for a minimum of five days or until drainage has ceased. The Foley catheter can be removed approximately 12 days postoperatively.

The primary advantage of radical perineal prostatectomy is that, if lymph node staging is not necessary, an abdominal incision is avoided and postoper-

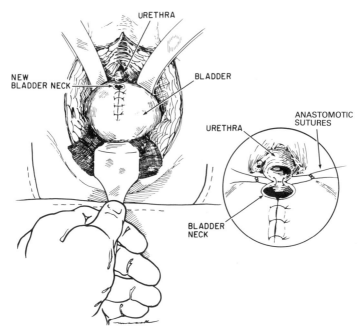

FIG 3–4.
Closure of bladder neck prior to vesicourethral anastomosis. Excellent exposure for the anastomosis is obtained by the perineal approach.

ative pulmonary complications may be decreased. No increased incidence of deep venous thrombosis has been identified despite the exaggerated lithotomy positioning. Blood loss is usually less than after radical retropubic prostatectomy, and excellent exposure for the vesicourethral anastomosis is obtained.

Radical Retropubic Prostatectomy

Radical retropubic prostatectomy is performed through an incision extending from the pubic symphysis to the umbilicus. Pelvic lymphadenectomy is completed first and frozen-section evaluation is performed. Depending upon the stage of the primary tumor, 5% to 10% of patients with grossly normal and histologically negative lymph nodes on frozen section will have microscopic tumor identified on permanent section evaluation of the lymph nodes. However, this incidence is low enough that a staged procedure wherein radical retropubic prostatectomy is performed after permanent sections of the lymph nodes are available is rarely indicated.

After the frozen-section report is obtained, radical retropubic prostatectomy is performed if the lymph nodes are histologically free of tumor. The bladder is mobilized from the pubic symphysis and the space of Retzius is exposed by blunt dissection. The bladder and prostate are retracted laterally from the pelvic side wall to expose the endopelvic fascia. Using a right-angle instrument, the endopelvic fascia is entered bluntly and the plane between the prostate and the pelvic side wall developed with finger dissection. Large veins course over the surface of the prostate in this area, so the incision in the endopelvic fascia should be made far enough laterally to prevent damage to this venous plexus.

After the endopelvic fascia has been incised bilaterally, the bladder and prostate are manually depressed posteriorly. The superficial branch of the dorsal vein of the penis is then encountered. A single, large vein is usually identifiable at this point and should be divided between absorbable ligatures. The vein is quite friable and easily avulsed, so care should be taken in applying the hemostatic ligature. The puboprostatic ligaments are then divided. These are identifiable as thick white bands of tissue connecting the anterior surface of the prostate to the pubis. They should be divided sharply with scissors at a point just below the pubis. The deep dorsal vein complex (Santorini's plexus) lies just behind the puboprostatic ligaments and anterior to the urethra. A right-angle clamp can be passed beneath this venous complex and anterior to the urethra.[10] A zero polyglycolic acid suture is then tied securely around the deep dorsal vein complex.

It is difficult to pass two ties around this complex that are sufficiently spaced so that division between ligatures is feasible. Therefore, after a single ligature is secured, the venous complex is divided sharply just cephalad to the ligature. Back bleeding from the prostate and bladder neck is controlled initially with manual pressure over a sponge until good hemostasis is obtained at the distal aspect. Hemostatic sutures are then placed in the anterior prostatic capsule to control the back bleeding.

Often, the maneuver described above does not result in complete hemostasis. Bleeding from the dorsal vein complex may occur during division of the puboprostatic ligaments or when the right-angle clamp is passed anterior to the urethra. Also, the hemostatic ligature that has been placed around the dorsal vein complex may become dislodged after the veins are divided because of the short stump distally. When this occurs, good hemostasis can be obtained by passage of a suture ligature of zero polyglycolic acid through the distal dorsal vein complex. Hemostasis must be relatively complete at this point of the operation before proceeding with the remainder of the surgery.

After the dorsal vein complex is secured, the urethra should be readily palpable (Fig 3–5). A right-angle clamp is passed around the urethra at the apex of the prostate. This maneuver is usually relatively easy, and care should be taken to include only the urethra in the clamp. The anterior portion of the urethra is divided sharply. The Foley catheter is then identified within the urethra and several centimeters of the distal catheter drawn into the incison. The catheter is then cut sharply distal to a large clamp. Superior traction on the catheter allows identification of the remainder of the posterior urethra which is divided sharply. Using Metzenbaum scissors, the rectourethralis muscle is then gently spread and cut just at the midline of the distal prostate. After these muscle attachments are severed, an index finger can be passed in the plane between Denonvilliers' fascia and the fat overlying the anterior rectal wall. The greatest risk of rectal injury occurs at this point, so care should be taken if the plane does not develop easily.

With a finger passed in the plane between the prostate and rectum, the lateral prostatic pedicle and neurovascular bundle are both palpable and visible. If sexual potency is not a concern the lateral pedicles can then be divided along both sides by passing a right-angle clamp in the space created by blunt dissection and using successive ligatures of absorbable 2–0 suture. Ligation of the prostatic pedicles bilaterally allows complete mobilization of the prostate and identification of the seminal vesicles and ampullary portion of the vasa deferentia.

Walsh and Mastwin[17] have described a technique for preservation of sexual potency during radical retropubic prostatectomy. If this approach is used, the operation proceeds in a manner identical to that described above until after the plane between the prostate and rectum is developed bluntly by finger dissection. The parasymphathetic nerves, which apparently are responsible for erectile function, course in the thin reflection of the endopelvic fascia onto the anterior surface of the prostate.[18] The nerves lie posterolateral to the urethra. They can be dissected free from the prostate and damage to the nerves avoided during ligation of the pedicle. The thin reflection of the endopelvic fascia onto the prostate is identified just at the apex of the prostate in the

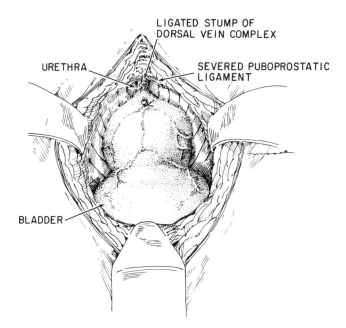

FIG 3–5.
Retropubic exposure of the prostate. The dorsal vein complex has been severed with ligatures. The prostatic apex and urethra are visualized. The neurovascular bundle responsible for erectile function lies posterolateral to the urethra.

posterolateral region when the urethra is divided. A right-angle clamp can be passed underneath this fascial layer, allowing its separation from the anterior capsule of the prostate. The fascia is divided anterior to the neurovascular bundle, which is then dissected laterally along with the fascial layer. This exposes the prostatic pedicle, which is secured in the manner described above.

After the entire prostatic pedicle has been divided, the mobilized distal prostate is then lifted superiorly using the previously divided distal end of the Foley catheter. An incision in the posterior layer of Denonvilliers' fascia is then made overlying the seminal vesicles and ampullary portion of the vasa deferentia. Five milliliters of indigo carmine should be administered intravenously at this point to facilitate identification of the ureteral orifices later. The vasa deferentia are divided sharply and the seminal vesicles dissected free in their entirety.

The prostate is then placed back in its anatomical position and the junction between the anterior prostatic capsule and the bladder neck is identified. Using an electrocautery, an incision is made in the anterior bladder neck just proximal to the prostate. The balloon on the Foley catheter is then deflated and the distal portion of the catheter brought through the incision in the anterior bladder neck and used for traction on the prostate. Small sponges are placed in the dome of the bladder. A small Deavor retractor placed within the bladder allows superior retraction and visualization of the bladder trigone. The incision along the lateral bladder wall to the trigone is continued using the electrocautery. The ureteral orifices are identified. Ureteral catheters may be placed at this point but are not mandatory if visualization is adequate. An incision is made through the trigone of the bladder, and the bladder base is undermined and mobilized for a short distance. Continuation of the dissection through the areolar and fibrous tissue overlying the seminal vesicles completes the dissection, and the specimen—consisting of the entire prostate and prostatic capsule as well as the seminal vesicles and ampullary portion of the vasa deferentia—is removed (Fig 3–6).

An alternative approach to radical retropubic prostatectomy is to perform prostatic removal proceeding in an antegrade fashion from the bladder neck to the urethra. This approach, described by Campbell,[19] has the potential advantage of early ligation of the vascular pedicle. In addition, division of the dorsal vein complex, often the portion of the procedure associated with the greatest blood loss, is reserved until the end. However, preservation of the lateral neurovascular bundle necessary for potency may be difficult with this approach.

After careful hemostasis is obtained, the bladder neck is closed in a posterior-to-anterior racket handle fashion using 2–0 absorbable sutures. Care should be taken to avoid incorporation of the ureteral orifices or ureters in this closure. The new bladder neck at the anterior portion of the incision should be large enough to admit a fingertip.

The vesicourethral anastomosis is now performed. Posterior displacement of the rectum using a malleable retractor placed over a sponge facilitates ex-

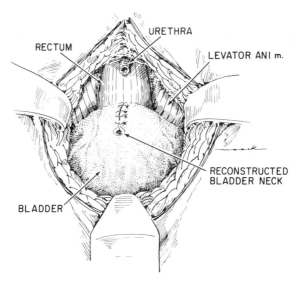

FIG 3–6.
After the specimen has been removed, bladder neck closure and vesicourethral anastomosis is performed.

posure of the urethra. A 20 French Foley catheter is placed through the penis and the distal end is visualized as it emerges through the urethra at the urogenital diaphragm; 2–0 absorbable sutures are used for the anastomosis. Placement of the sutures through the urethra should be completed first. The tip of the needle is placed in contact with the end of the Foley catheter. The catheter is then slowly withdrawn into the urethra, guiding the needle. Mucosa should be included in the urethral sutures. Usually, six sutures are placed, all passing inside the urethra to out. The sutures are then tagged accordingly with appropriate clamps. A needle is then threaded onto the end of the suture which is inside the urethra and the sutures are placed in corresponding positions on the bladder neck. A zero polypropylene suture is passed through the eye of the Foley catheter. Both ends of this suture are then passed through a straight needle, which is passed through the bladder neck and out the dome of the bladder. This suture is used later to secure the Foley catheter to a button placed on the anterior abdominal wall as a backup in case the Foley balloon should burst. The Foley catheter is passed into the bladder and the balloon inflated with 10 ml of fluid. Slight traction is then used to position the bladder neck, and the anastomotic sutures are tied securely. The Foley catheter is irrigated to ensure its optimal positioning and to check the integrity of the anastomosis. Penrose drains are brought out through a stab wound in a lower quadrant of the abdomen, and the incision is closed with interrupted No. 1 polyglycolic acid sutures. The previously placed prolene suture is tied loosely over a button just lateral to the incision.

Postoperatively, nasogastric suction is not necessary on a routine basis, and patient feeding begins as soon as postoperative ileus resolves. Early ambulation is important. Patients usually are discharged within a week and the Foley catheter removed approximately 12 days after surgery.

Complications

Patients undergoing radical prostatectomy are subject to the same potential complications as any major pelvic operation. However, the incidence of wound infection, deep venous thrombosis, cardiovascular, or pulmonary complications is relatively low. Intraoperative blood loss averages 600 to 1,200 ml and generally is somewhat less with the perineal approach. Excessive intraoperative blood loss can be avoided by careful and anatomical control of the deep dorsal vein complex.

The other complications discussed below are those that may be somewhat peculiar to radical prostatectomy or that occur with sufficient frequency that they require specific mention.

Urinary Incontinence

Perhaps the most feared complication of radical prostatectomy is urinary incontinence. Incontinence is reported to have occurred in from 0 to more than 50% of patients who have undergone radical prostatectomy. A realistic figure is that approximately 5% of patients will have significant postoperative incontinence, whereas another 15% to 20% will experience minor to moderate stress incontinence.[20, 21] Therefore, the substantial majority of patients can be expected to regain good urinary control.

Several technical points may be important in preservation of continence. Since the effect of any internal sphincteric mechanism at the bladder neck as well as the intrinsic tone of the prostate is lost postoperatively, urinary continence relies to a great extent on the external sphincter. Therefore, division of the urethra should be at the level of the prostatic apex, and anastomotic sutures should exclude the sphincteric mechanism. In addition, excessive removal of bladder neck tissue may compromise return of any intrinsic sphincteric mechanism of the bladder neck.

Return of urinary control after radical prostatectomy is a gradual process. The substantial majority of patients have regained relatively good control within two to three months of surgery, although the ultimate potential for recovery may not be realized until nine months to a year postoperatively. Modest amounts of stress incontinence may be treated satisfactorily by sympathomimetic drugs such as ephedrine sulphate or bladder antispasmodics such as oxybutynin. If more marked urinary incontinence is persistent, insertion of an inflatable artificial urinary sphincter can be highly successful.

Impotence

Previously, the incidence of erectile impotence after radical prostatectomy exceeded 90%. In 1982, Walsh and Donker[22] described the pelvic anatomy of the parasympathetic nervous system and identified the nerves that appear to be responsible for potency. A technique was developed in which the neuro-vascular bundle containing these nerves could be preserved (see above). Walsh and Mastwin[17] have reported a postoperative potency rate in excess of 90% using this technique. Although others have had difficulty reproducing potency rates this high, it seems reasonable to anticipate that approximately half of the patients with no problems with sexual potency preoperatively can retain erectile function postoperatively if this technique is used.

In a significant number of patients, sexual function is diminished or absent prior to surgery. For these patients, as well as for many others, sexual function is not an issue and radical prostatectomy should be performed without efforts to preserve the parasympathetic neurovascular bundle. Concerns have been expressed that the potency-sparing approach to radical prostatectomy may result in inadequate margins. In general, removal of the thin reflection of endopelvic fascia with the potency sparing approach does not compromise the procedure or violate the principles of cancer surgery.[18] However, if potency is not a concern, wider ligation of the vascular pedicles and sacrifice of the neuro-vascular bundle seem logical.

Rectal Injury

Intraoperative rectal injury occurs in 1% to 2% of patients undergoing radical prostatectomy. The incidence may be slightly increased with radical perineal prostatectomy. Also, previous pelvic irradiation or a prior transurethral resection of the prostate may produce periprostatic fibrosis and some difficulty separating the prostate from the rectum. The greatest risk of rectal injury during either the perineal or retropubic approach is when the rectourethralis muscle is divided. After this, the rectum falls away from the prostate and can be retracted from harm.

If contamination is not excessive and the rectal laceration is relatively regular and identifiable, multiple layer primary closure and copious irrigation along with postoperative antibiotics are sufficient in most patients. However, performance of a proximal diverting colostomy may be prudent.

Prostatorectal fistula may result if an intraoperative rectal laceration occurs. A diverting colostomy along with catheter drainage of the bladder may allow spontaneous closure of some prostatorectal fistulas. If the fistula is persistent, a modified York-Mason approach has given excellent results with minimal morbidity.[23] Using this procedure, direct posterior access to the fistula is obtained and multiple layer closure can be performed (Fig 3–7). Colostomy has not been necessary if an elemental diet is maintained for one to two weeks postoperatively.

Anastomotic Stricture

Strictures at the vesicourethral anastomosis occur in a small percentage of patients and may result in postoperative incontinence or voiding difficulty. Technical factors probably contribute to most anastomotic strictures. A careful approximation of the mucosa is of greatest importance in preventing strictures, and care should be taken to include only the urethra in the anastomotic su-

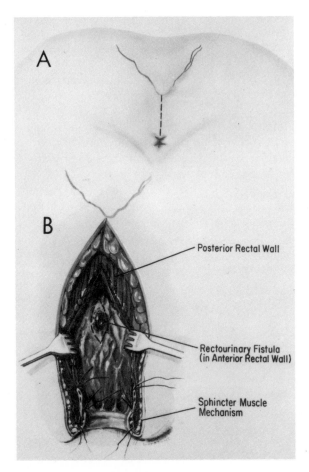

FIG 3–7.
A, diagram showing incision for modified York-Mason repair of prostatorectal fistula. A linear incision is made between the posterior anal verge and the coccyx. Patients are placed in a prone jackknife position. **B,** division of the rectal sphincter and posterior rectal wall allows direct access and repair of the rectourinary fistula with excellent visualization.

tures. Strictures can usually be managed adequately with dilation. The Vest technique for vesicourethral anastomosis, in which buttressing sutures between the bladder neck and perineum are used, may be associated with a higher incidence of postoperative stricture.

RADIATION THERAPY

Although some form of ionizing radiation has been used as treatment of prostatic cancers for over 60 years, widespread use of radiation for definitive therapy of prostatic cancer did not occur until the 1960s. Several factors led to renewed interest in radiation treatment of prostatic cancer, primarily the development of cobalt 60 radiation sources as well as linear accelerators. The use of interstitial implantation of radioactive isotopes such as iodine-125 or gold 198 was initiated in the early 1970s, and afterloading of iridium 192 was described in the late 1970s. Most recently, electron beam therapy has been used.

External Irradiation

Orthovoltage irradiation initially found limited acceptance as a treatment for prostatic cancer primarily because of the damage to skin and subcutaneous tissue that occurred when potentially lethal doses were delivered to prostatic cancer cells. Cobalt 60 units and, more recently, linear accelerators allow delivery of potentially lethal doses of radiation with less fibrosis and radiation damage to skin.

The total dose of radiation is a balance between the amount required for elimination of viable tumor cells and the tolerance of normal tissues. For palpable prostate cancers, a dose of 6,500 to 7,000 rad should be delivered to the prostate itself,[24] while lower doses (4,500 to 5,000 rad) may be sufficient for microscopic disease in periprostatic tissues. For the urinary bladder, a dose of 5,000 rad presents a 5% probability of radiation injury, while 8,000 rad results in a 50% probability of permanent radiation damage.[25]

Not all tissues are equally sensitive to radiation. Several factors that are highly unquantifiable and unpredictable, such as the half-life of tumor cells and the degree of hypoxia, may have profound effects upon the ability of cells to repair DNA damage produced by ionizing irradiation. The concept of fractionation of radiation doses arose from the recognition that complications could be reduced and, perhaps, efficacy improved by multiple applications of fractionated doses of radiation. Normal tissues are able to tolerate fractionated doses better. In addition, fractionation of the dose may allow delivery of radiation to more tumor cells at a point at which they are most sensitive to the toxic effects of radiation.

Technique

Recognition of some of these proven and theoretical biologic factors of radiation-induced tissue injury has led to adoption of the treatment schemes most commonly in use today. There is no uniformity of opinion regarding the optimal technique for delivery of external irradiation for prostatic cancer. In addition, availability of equipment and experience of the radiation therapist vary. Finally, ongoing research and clinical studies are attempting to define the optimal regimens for radiation treatment of prostatic cancer. Nevertheless, the technique described here is one that follows, at least in general, the guidelines for most current treatment plans for delivery of potentially curative doses of external beam irradiation in patients with prostatic cancer.

Some treatment plans still use cobalt 60, a synthetic isotope that emits protons with an energy around 1.25 million electron volts (meV). More often,

4 to 6 meV linear accelerators are used as an energy source for treatment of prostatic cancer. The energy beam from a linear accelerator can be focused more precisely. Treatment morbidity from damage to normal structures is reduced using linear accelerators.

The portal size and total dose is of critical importance in determining treatment outcome and subsequent complications (Fig 3–8). The maximal dose of radiation that can be delivered to the tumor without producing permanent damage to normal tissues is desirable. As discussed in chapter 6, there seems little reason to use radiation portals that encompass the whole pelvis since no therapeutic benefit has been demonstrated in patients with pelvic lymph node metastasis. However, some radiation therapists use portals that encompass the primary lymph node drainage of the pelvis and deliver a subsequent boost to the prostate. Most commonly, an isocentric technique with rotating fields is used. For simulation, x-ray films of the pelvis are obtained and the portals are marked with an indelible ink on the skin. The isocenter is similarly marked. In patients with palpable extracapsular extension, CT scans may be used to identify more accurately the volume of tissue to be irradiated.

In general, when the pelvic lymph nodes are treated, doses of 4,500 to 5,000 rad are delivered with a boost to the prostate. Fractionation of the dose usually extends the treatment period to six to eight weeks. Portals that encompass the entire prostate and periprostatic region should be used, and this gen-

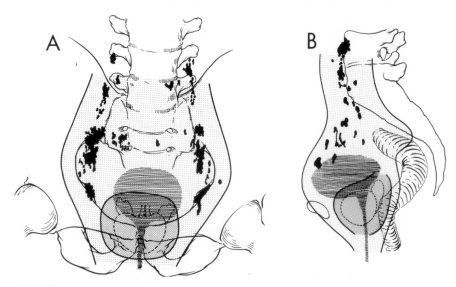

FIG 3–8.
Schematic representation of the radiation therapy portals used for prostatic carcinoma employing a four-field treatment technique. The lightly stippled area is treated with 5,000 rad and the smaller, heavily stippled area is boosted to 7,000 rad. Regional lymph nodes opacified by lymphangiography are shown in black. **A,** volume encompassed by opposed anterior and posterior beams. **B,** lateral projection showing the area encompassed by opposed lateral beams. (Reproduced with permission from the *Annual Review of Medicine,* vol 33, 1981, by Annual Reviews, Inc.)

erally requires fields of at least 9 × 9 cm. The actual field size varies depending upon the patient size but should extend from the ischial tuberosities to the fifth lumbar vertebra in an AP dimension. Laterally, the treatment portals cover the area between the anterior portion of the prostate and the middle half of the rectal lumen.

Complications of External Irradiation

The efficacy of ionizing radiation in the treatment of cancer depends upon irreversible damage to tumor cells. However, normal cells are also subject to the lethal effects of ionizing radiation. Much of the acute injury caused by radiation is ultimately repaired, resulting in a lower incidence of chronic complications compared to acute side effects. In general, the side effects of external irradiation delivered for treatment of prostatic cancer are limited to pelvic organs located within the treatment fields, primarily the bladder, small bowel, and rectum. The incidence of complications is directly related to total dose, radiation portals, fractionation scheme, and the energy source.

Radiation Cystitis.—Acute radiation cystitis, manifested by urinary frequency, urgency, and nocturia, occurs in approximately 40% of patients. Hematuria, either microscopic or gross, may also be seen. Symptoms of acute radiation cystitis may occasionally be severe and are a cause for treatment interruption in 5% to 10% of patients. In the majority of patients, symptoms resolve within three months of therapy.

Chronic, symptomatic radiation cystitis occurs in about 10% of patients receiving curative doses of external irradiation.[26] The incidence of chronic cystitis is decreased if radiation portals are designed that encompass only the prostate and periprostatic region and exclude the remainder of the bladder. Chronic radiation cystitis is characterized by persistent frequency, urgency, and dysuria. Cystoscopically, the bladder has a typical appearance of pale mucosa with telangiectatic vessels on the surface. Bladder antispasmodics may provide symptomatic relief. Around 1% or 2% of patients develop a contracted bladder, and bladder augmentation or supravesical urinary diversion may be necessary.

Urethral Injury.—Urethral damage, resulting in urethral stricture and/or urinary incontinence, occurs in approximately 5% to 8% of patients after external irradiation. Radiation-induced urethral strictures may be particularly refractory to successful management by dilation or urethrotomy. Urinary incontinence occurs primarily in patients who have undergone a previous transurethral prostatectomy. Incontinence is reported to occur in 5% to 8% of patients after radiation treatment. Insertion of an inflatable urethral sphincter may be helpful with incontinence. However, many of the same patients have problems with urethral strictures, radiation cystitis, or both.

Gastrointestinal Complications.—Radiation enteritis resulting in diarrhea, anorexia, and nausea occurs primarily in patients receiving radiation to large pelvic fields. About 40% of patients in whom significant amounts of small bowel are included in the radiation field develop symptomatic acute radiation enteritis.[27] Symptoms resolve in most patients within three months, but around 10% have persistent, chronic symptoms, primarily diarrhea, related to radiation enteritis.

Radiation proctitis may also result in acute symptoms of diarrhea and, in some patients, rectal bleeding. Rectal stricture or fistula requiring a diverting colostomy is rare.

Impotence.—Slightly more than half of patients with normal sexual function before treatment retain their sexual potency after definitive doses of external irradiation for prostatic cancer. Whether this figure is improved by more limited fields and different dose fractionation is uncertain. Using gonadal shields, the dose of radiation delivered to the testes is enough to suppress germinal function but not Leydig cell secretion of testosterone. Presumably, radiation-induced impotence results from damage to small vessels and, either directly from the radiation or indirectly from ischemia, to parasympathetic nerves.

Interstitial Irradiation

Compared to external radiation sources, interstitial implantation of radioactive substances (brachytherapy) into the prostate has the potential advantage of delivering a higher dose of ionizing radiation to the prostate itself while limiting the effect on adjacent organs. Also, the long half-life of some isotopes theoretically may be of advantage in treating tumors with long doubling times. Primarily, three different isotopes have been used to treat prostatic cancer: iodine 125 (I 125), gold 198 (Au 198), and iridium 192 (Ir 192). Each has distinct energy specifications and effects upon prostatic cancer.

I 125 Implantation

The use of interstitial implantation of iodine 125 for treatment of prostatic cancer was initiated and popularized at Memorial Sloan-Kettering Cancer Center in the early 1970s.[30] The rationale for the use of iodine 125 was based upon the long half-life of the isotope coupled with the relatively low energy. Thus, high doses of radiation could be delivered to the prostate over a prolonged period while the adjacent structures received more limited amounts. In addition, it was believed that a larger number of patients would be potential candidates for iodine 125 implantation compared to radical prostatectomy.

Iodine 125 emits pure gamma radiation with a half-life of around 60 days. Thus, the useful life of the isotope or the period for which effective doses of radiation may be emitted is one year. The relatively low energy of iodine 125 along with the long half-life increase the safety and ease with which personnel can handle the isotope. The half value layer in tissue is only 1.7 cm. This factor limits the amount of radiation delivered to the rectum and bladder when the seeds are implanted in the prostate.

An iodine 125 seed consists of an outer shell of titanium. Enclosed within is the iodine 125 isotope absorbed on an ion-exchange resin. The emitted energy from the isotopes used in a particular operation varies somewhat and depends upon the shelf life or storage time of the isotope since some decay occurs with time. In general, seeds with an emitted energy between 0.45 keV and 5.5 keV are used. The targeted area of irradiation, that is, the entire prostate and tumor volume, should receive a minimum of 18,000 rad over the life of the isotope (one year) and an average dose of 25,000 rad. Comparison of doses of radiation delivered by brachytherapy to those with conventional fractionation schemes is difficult and, to a great extent, inaccurate. However, it is believed that the doses of radiation delivered by iodine 125 brachytherapy are roughly equivalent to around 7,000 rad of external beam irradiation delivered by conventional fractionation over seven weeks.

The geometry of the implant is important and a relatively uniform distribution of the seeds within the prostate and the tumor is attempted. Postoperative computerized dosimetry analysis should be performed to determine the isodose curves. The 16,000-rad curves should encompass the entire prostate and tumor volume. Although seed geometry is important, the low energy of the isotope generally creates relatively uniform isodose curves. The rectum and bladder usually fall well outside the 16,000-rad curve and often receive less than 4,000 rad of brachytherapy (Fig 3–9).

Patient Selection.—Originally, patients with clinical stage A, B, C, or D1 tumors were considered to be good candidates for treatment with iodine 125 implantation. Subsequent experience has led to more stringent selection criteria and identified groups of patients most likely to benefit from the opera-

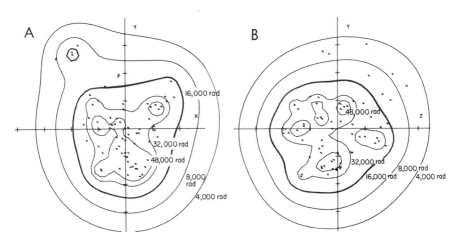

FIG 3–9.
A, computerized dosimetry analysis after iodine 125 implantation of the prostate. The prostate and tumor volume should receive a minimum dose of 16,000 rad over the life of the isotope. Doses to the rectum and bladder are substantially less. **B,** lateral view of computerized dosimetry analysis of prostate after iodine 125 implantation.

tion.[30] In patients with stage D1 disease, interstitial implantation represents a form of local therapy for what is likely a systemic disease. An initial analysis by Barzell and associates[31] indicated that patients with minimal volume nodal disease had a survival after iodine 125 implantation of the prostate and pelvic node dissection equivalent to that of patients with negative pelvic lymph nodes.

Susequent analysis has, however, confirmed the poor prognostic implication of any nodal metastases.[32] If positive pelvic lymph nodes are identified at the time of surgery, the decision to proceed with interstitial implantation of iodine 125 may be justified in some patients based upon the prospects for local tumor control and the low morbidity of the procedure. However, no survival benefit is likely to be imparted by the operation.

Patients with stage A carcinoma generally are poor condidates for interstitial implantation of iodine 125 seeds. The transurethral or open prostatectomy—which, by definition, all patients with stage A prostatic cancer have undergone—removes a substantial portion of the prostatic tissue. The remaining prostatic capsule and residual prostatic tissue usually are insufficient to support the seeds and allow a good geometric distribution.

Since a relatively uniform geometric and anatomical distribution of the seeds is desirable, definition of tumor extent by digital palpation is mandatory. Therefore, patients with any other than minor amounts of extracapsular tumor extension probably are better treated by alternative methods such as external irradiation. As would be expected, the best results after iodine 125 implantation of prostatic cancer have been obtained in patients with intracapsular, relatively well-differentiated tumors, but 16,000 rad isodose curves that encompass small amounts of extracapsular extension are possible.

Technique.—Patients are placed in a modified lithotomy position which allows transrectal digital palpation of the prostate to be performed intraoperatively. A midline incision is made from umbilicus to pubis and a bilateral pelvic lymph node dissection is performed. The endopelvic fascia is incised bilaterally and the prostate bluntly mobilized from the lateral pelvic wall. The dorsal vein of the penis is ligated, but it is not necessary to take down the puboprostatic ligaments.

After retropubic exposure of the prostate is obtained in this fashion, a finger is inserted into the rectum and an 18-gauge needle 15 cm in length is passed through the anterior capsule of the prostate just lateral to the urethra. The rectal finger palpates the tip of the needle as it penetrates the posterior capsule; the needle tip is then withdrawn to a point within the posterior capsule. The prostatic volume is then calculated by measuring the three dimensions of the prostate. The portion of the needle protruding from the prostate is measured by a ruler and subtracted from the 15-cm length of the needle to determine the anterior/posterior dimension. The length and width of the prostate are then measured directly and the volume determined. A designed nomogram is then used to determine the number of seeds necessary and the spacing between needles (Fig 3–10).

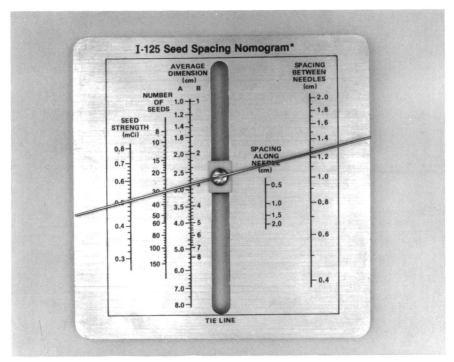

FIG 3–10.
Nomogram used for determining number of iodine 125 seeds required for optimal dosimetry. A tie line connects the seed strength with the average dimension of the prostate to determine the number of seeds required.

Depending on the prostatic size, around three seeds are implanted per needle. An appropriate number of needles are then inserted throughout the prostate with the depth of insertion determined by the rectal finger. The needles should be distributed fairly uniformly throughout the prostate, although with a tendency toward a greater concentration of needles on the side of the tumor. Care should be taken to include the entire periphery of the tumor volume and prostate.

After the needles have been inserted, the seeds are loaded into the needles with a modified application device (Fig 3–11). The seeds are spaced between ½ and 1 cm apart along the needle track, then the needle is withdrawn. After the needles have all been removed, a detection device is used to check the suction and any sponges used during surgery so that stray seeds can be recovered. Hemostatic sutures of 2–0 chromic occasionally are necessary at needle puncture sites. After good hemostasis has been obtained, a Penrose drain is inserted and the incision closed. The Foley catheter is removed on the second postoperative day. Hospital discharge usually occurs on about the fifth day postoperatively.

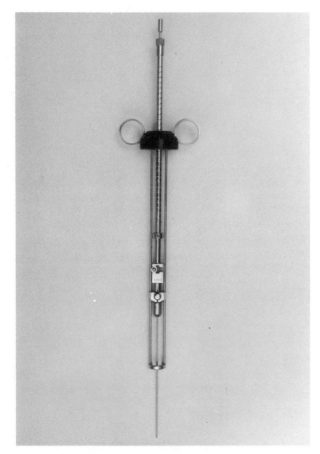

FIG 3–11.
Modified apparatus for insertion of iodine 125 seeds. The needle is grasped and the inserter used to place the seeds within the substance of the prostate.

Complications.—One of the primary advantages of the use of iodine 125 isotopes in the treatment of prostatic cancer is the generally low morbidity associated with the procedure. The relatively low doses of irradiation delivered to adjacent organs decrease complications.

Urinary Complications.—Irritative voiding symptoms consisting of urgency, frequency, and dysuria occur in about half the patients immediately after catheter removal but generally resolve within one week of treatment. Voiding symptoms persisting longer than three months occur in approximately 5% of patients.

Management of obstructive voiding symptoms both preoperatively and postoperatively deserves special comment. If a relatively complete transurethral prostatectomy is performed preoperatively, the residual prostatic tissue may be insufficient for implantation of iodine 125 seeds. On the other hand, a certain degree of inflammation and prostatic edema from the acute radiation injury can be expected postoperatively, and patients may have increased symptoms or develop urinary retention within several months after the procedure if obstructive tissue is not removed.

In the Memorial Hospital series, limited transurethral prostatectomy and iodine 125 implantation have been performed as staged procedures to allow the prostatic fossa to reepithelialize before implantation of the radioactive seeds. In 47 patients, we have performed a limited resection of the prostate followed immediately by implantation of iodine 125 seeds. No complications have resulted from this approach. All patients have been able to void satisfactorily postoperatively, and there have been no patients with prolonged irritative voiding symptoms or recognized problems related to this approach. An average of 5 gm of prostatic tissue has been removed. During the resection, only the central portion of the obstructive tissue should be removed. Care should be taken to prevent undermining of the lateral lobes, which could require resection of larger volumes of tissue.

If at all possible, transurethral prostatectomy should be avoided during the first year after surgery. Some of the seeds necessary for delivery of effective doses of irradiation may be removed with the prostatic tissue, and a prolonged healing period may ensue because of the ongoing radiation damage. The titanium sheath of the seed causes an electrical short when an arc is created with the electrocautery. While this presents no danger to the patient or surgeon, the cutting effect of the electrocautery is lost temporarily, and contact between the cautery loop and the seed must be discontinued before the cutting effect is restored.

Rectal Complications.—Usually, the dose of irradiation delivered to the rectum is relatively minimal. However, some patients develop localized areas of radiation proctitis. This may be manifested by diarrhea or rectal pain as well as some rectal bleeding. Prostatorectal fistula occurs in less than 1% of patients. The incidence of rectal complications including fistula is increased when supplemental external irradiation is delivered after iodine 125 implantation.[33]

Effects on Sexual Potency.—One of the principle advantages of iodine 125 implantation in the treatment of prostatic cancer is that sexual potency is preserved in the majority of patients. Over 90% of patients who are sexually active before therapy maintain their potency after the procedure.[34] In most patients, loss of sexual potency has been reported as an early postoperative event, and the relation to the radiation itself is uncertain.

Interstitial Au 198

Interstitial implantation of Au 198 isotopes in the prostate along with supplemental external beam irradiation as treatment of localized prostatic cancer was developed by Carlton and colleagues[35] in 1972 and has been used primarily at Baylor University. Au 198 has properties that present advantages and disadvantages. Both beta and gamma irradiation are emitted from Au 198, and the half value layer in tissue is 4.5 cm. Au 198 has a relatively short half-life of less than three days. Therefore, the useful life of the isotope is approximately three weeks (compared to one year with iodine 125).

The relatively high energy of Au 198 requires protection for personnel involved with its use. However, geometric placement of seeds is not critical because of the high energy. The half-life of 2.7 days decreases the shelf life of the isotope but allows subsequent delivery of adjuvant external beam irradiation.

Au 198 seeds are used primarily to deliver a boost dose of irradiation to the prostate, and supplemental external irradiation is used after the radiation energy from the Au 198 seeds is exhausted. Since the procedure only requires implantation of some six to ten seeds, patients with a previous transurethral resection are considered candidates for the procedure. Thus, the operation is applicable to patients with stage A tumors, stage B tumors, and small stage C lesions.

Technique.—A pelvic lymphadenectomy is performed through either a lower midline incision or a lower transverse abdominal incision as is described at Baylor University. After lymphadenectomy, retropubic exposure of the prostate is obtained. Depending upon tumor size, anywhere from six to ten seeds with an average strength of 30 to 40 mCi are implanted in the prostate.[36] A greater number of seeds are implanted in the tumor nodule itself. Approximately 3,000 rad of irradiation are delivered to the implanted volume and surrounding periprostatic tissue over the useful life of the isotope, i.e., about three weeks.

Supplemental external irradiation is delivered at least three weeks after the implant. Survival rates in patients with positive pelvic lymph nodes have been disappointing, and pelvic external irradiation generally is not useful in this setting. However, if lymph nodes are free of metastases, 4,500 rad are delivered at fractionated doses of 250 rad/day. The portals encompass the prostate and periprostatic tissue only and exclude the pelvic lymph nodes.

Complications.—The only large series of patients available for review and determination of complications originates from Baylor University.[36] Twelve percent of patients were reported to have symptoms of radiation proctitis acutely, but persistent symptoms were only seen in 4% of patients. Prolonged symptoms of radiation cystitis were seen in around 3% of patients, and treatment-related erectile impotence was recognized in approximately one third of patients treated.

Iridium 192

Iridium 192 emits gamma energy. The half-life of the isotope is 75 days and the half value layer in tissue is 6 cm. The technique for implantation of iridium 192 involves afterloading of needles placed intraoperatively.[37] Patients are placed in a lithotomy position and a pelvic lymphadenectomy is performed. The prostate is visualized through the abdominal incision, and 18 needles of 17-gauge size are positioned using a perineal template. Afterloading of the iridium 192 decreases the radiation hazard for personnel. Postoperatively, the temporary lead wires are removed from the needles and the iridium 192 is inserted. The iridium 192 needles are left in place for some 40 to 50 hours and then removed. Three thousand to 3,500 rad are delivered to the prostate and periprostatic tissue over this period. Some two weeks later, supplemental external irradiation is delivered to 8 × 8 cm portals.

The experience with interstitial irradiation using Ir 192 either alone or in combination with external irradiation as treatment of prostatic cancer is limited. Early results show good local control rates. However, rectal complications including fistula have been reported, and urinary incontinence or urethral stricture is also possible. In Miller's series of 14 patients who received 2,000 rad of external beam therapy prior to 5,000 rad of interstitial irradiation using iridium 192, rectal complications requiring colostomy occurred in two patients.[38]

CRYOSURGERY

Cryosurgery for treatment of prostatic cancer has been used primarily at the University of Iowa. Originally, it was thought that antibodies against prostatic cancer could be induced by the process of cryotherapy and that the procedure may have indications in patients with metastatic disease.[39] Subsequent analysis of treatment results as well as immunologic studies have shown no evidence that any immune response is elicited by cryodestruction of the prostate.

Cryosurgery is rarely used today. Local recurrence as high as 60% has been documented in the absence of early endocrine therapy. In addition, urinary incontinence has been reported to occur in 15% of patients, fecal incontinence in 2%, and urethrocutaneous fistula in 7%.[40]

LASER SURGERY

The use of lasers in the treatment of prostatic cancer has been limited to application of a neodymium:YAG laser in patients with stage A carcinoma. In the technique described by Sander and Beisland,[41] the laser fiber is inserted into the prostatic fossa through a trocar cystoscope. Using a power output of 45 to 50 watts, the residual prostatic capsule is thermally coagulated with laser energy. Easiest access is to the posterior capsule. No treatment complications were observed in the initial 16 patients treated. In particular, there was no incidence of laser injury to the rectum.

The efficacy of this treatment cannot be determined because of the short follow-up. However, the 1,060-nm wavelength of a neodymium:YAG laser produces thermal coagulation for a maximum depth of 4 to 6 mm. Whether this is sufficient for complete destruction of the prostatic capsule and any residual cancer and how uniformly this can be distributed remain to be determined.

McPhee and colleagues[42] have reported interstitial implantation of fibers from an argon-dye laser in the Dunning rat tumor model. The animals are first photosensitized with hematoporphyrin derivative and 630-nm light delivered. Tumor regression has been observed, but the procedure has not been performed clinically.

REFERENCES

1. Jewett HJ, Bridge RW, Gray GF Jr, et al: The palpable nodule of prostatic cancer. *JAMA* 1968; 203:115–118.
2. Hodges CV, Pearse HD, Stille L: Radical prostatectomy for carcinoma: 30-year experience and 15-year survivals. *J Urol* 1979; 122:180–182.
3. Schroeder FH, Belt E: Carcinoma of the prostate: A study of 213 patients with stage C tumors treated by total perineal prostatectomy. *J Urol* 1975; 114:257–260.
4. Zincke H, Utz DC: Radical surgery for stage D1 prostatic cancer. *Semin Urol* 1983; 4:253–260.
5. Catalona WJ, Kadmon D, Crane DB: Effect of minidose heparin on lymphocele formation following extraperitoneal pelvic lymphadenectomy. *J Urol* 1980; 123:890–892.
6. Dahl DS, Wilson CS, Middleton RG, et al: Pelvic lymphadenectomy for staging localized prostatic cancer. *J Urol* 1974; 112:245–246.
7. Catalona WJ, Stein AJ: Staging errors in clinically localized prostatic cancer. *J Urol* 1982; 127:452–456.
8. Sogani PC, Watson RC, Whitmore WF, Jr: Lymphocele after pelvic lymphadenectomy for urologic cancer. *Urology* 1981; 17:39–43.
9. Paulson DF: The prognostic role of lymphadenectomy in adenocarcinoma of the prostate. *Urol Clin North Am* 1980; 7:615–622.
10. Young HH: The early diagnosis and radical cure of carcinoma of the prostate: Being a study of 40 cases and presentation of a radical operation which was carried out in 4 cases. *Bull Johns Hopkins Hosp* 1905; 16:315–321.
11. Millen T: *Retropubic Urinary Surgery*. Baltimore, Williams & Wilkins Co, 1947.
12. Walsh PC, Lepor H, Eggleston JC: Radical prostatectomy with preservation of sexual function: Anatomical and pathologic considerations. *Prostate* 1983; 4:473–485.
13. Smith JA Jr, Seaman JP, Gleidman JB, et al: Pelvic lymph node metastases from prostatic cancer: Influence of tumor grade and stage in 452 consecutive patients. *J Urol* 1983; 130:290–292.
14. Belt E, Ebert CE, Surber AC Jr: A new anatomic approach in perineal prostatectomy. *J Urol* 1939; 41:482–497.
15. Hodges CV: Vesicourethral anastomosis after radical prostatectomy: Experience with the Jewett modification. *J Urol* 1977; 118:209–210.
16. Reiner WG, Walsh PC: An anatomical approach to the surgical management of the dorsal vein and Santorini's plexus during radical retropubic surgery. *J Urol* 1979; 121:198–200.

17. Walsh PC, Mastwin JL: Radical prostatectomy and cystoprostatectomy with preservation of potency: Results utilizing a new nerve sparing technique. *Br J Urol* 1984; 56:694–697.

18. Lepor H, Gregerman M, Crosby R, et al: Precise localization of the autonomic nerves from the pelvic plexus to the corpora cavernosa: A detailed anatomical study of the adult male pelvis. *J Urol* 1985; 133:207–212.

19. Campbell EW: Total prostatectomy with preliminary ligation of the vascular pedicles. *J Urol* 1959; 81:464–467.

20. Smith JA, Jr, Middleton RG: Radical prostatectomy for stage B_2 prostatic cancer. *J Urol* 1982; 127:702–703.

21. Boxer RJ, Kaufman JJ, Goodwin WE: Radical prostatectomy for carcinoma of the prostate, 1951–1976: A review of 329 patients. *J Urol* 1977; 117:208–213.

22. Walsh PC, Donker PJ: Impotence following radical prostatectomy: Insight into etiology and prevention. *J Urol* 1982; 128:492–497.

23. Dahl DS, Howard PM, Middleton RG: Surgical management of recto-urinary fistula. *J Urol* 1974; 111:514–517.

24. Hanks GE, Leibel SA, Krall JM, et al: Patterns of care studies: Dose response observation for local control of adenocarcinoma of the prostate. *Int J Radiol Oncol Biol Phys* 1985; 11:153–157.

25. Stewart JR, Gibbs FA, Jr: Prevention of radiation injury. *Ann Rev Med* 1982; 33:385–395.

26. Ray GR, Cassady R, Bagshaw MA: Definitive radiation therapy of carcinoma of the prostate: A report on 15 years of experience. *Radiology* 1973; 106:407–418.

27. Perez CA, Bauer W, Garza R, et al: Radiation therapy in the treatment of localized carcinoma of the prostate. *Cancer* 1974; 34:1059–1068.

28. Bagshaw MA, Ray GR, Pistenma DA, et al: External beam radiation therapy of primary carcinoma of the prostate. *Cancer* 1975; 36:723–728.

29. Whitmore WF Jr, Hilaris B, Grabstald H: Retropubic implantation of iodine 125 in the treatment of prostatic cancer. *J Urol* 1972; 108:918–920.

30. Whitmore WF Jr: Interstitial radiation therapy for carcinoma of the prostate. *Prostate* 1980; 1:157–168.

31. Barzell W, Bean MA, Hilaris BS, et al: Prostatic adenocarcinoma: Relationship of grade and local extent to the pattern of metastases. *J Urol* 1977; 118:278–282.

32. Grossman HB, Batata M, Hilaris B, et al: I-125 implantation for carcinoma of the prostate: Further follow-up of first 100 cases. *Urology* 1982; 20:591–598.

33. DeVere White R, Babaian RK, Feldman M, et al: Adjunctive therapy with interstitial irradiation for prostate cancer. *Urology* 1982; 19:395–398.

34. Herr HW: Preservation of sexual potency in prostatic cancer patients after pelvic lymphadenectomy and retropubic I-125 implantation. *J Urol* 1979; 121:621–623.

35. Carlton CE Jr, Dawoud F, Hudgins P, et al: Irradiation treatment of carcinoma of the prostate: A preliminary report based on 8 years of experience. *J Urol* 1972; 108:924–927.

36. Scardino PT, Guerriero WG, Carlton CE Jr: Surgical staging and combined therapy with radioactive gold groin implantation and external irradiation, in Johnson DE, Boileau MA (eds): *Genitourinary tumors: Fundamental principles and surgical techniques.* New York, Grune & Stratton, 1982, pp 75–90.

37. Tansey LA, Shanberg AM, Syed AM, et al: Treatment of prostatic carcinoma by pelvic lymphadenectomy, and temporary iridium 192 implant and external irradiation. *Urology* 1983; 21:594–598.

38. Miller LS: Afterloading transperineal iridium-192 wire implantation of the prostate. *Radiology* 1979; 13:527–528.

39. Gonder MH, Soanes WA, Smith V: Experimental prostate cryosurgery. *Invest Urol* 1964; 1:610–619.

40. Bonney WW, Fallon B, Gerber WL, et al: Cryosurgery in prostatic cancer: Elimination of the local lesion. *Urology* 1983; 22:8–15.

41. Sander S, Beisland HO: Laser in the treatment of localized prostatic carcinoma. *J Urol* 1984; 132:280–281.

42. McPhee MS, Thorndyke CW, Thomas G, et al: Interstitial applications of laser irradiation in hemoatoporphyrin derivative photosensitized Dunning R3327 prostate cancers. *Lasers Surg Med* 1984; 4:93–98.

4

Stage A Carcinoma of the Prostate

Although tumors are often described as "clinical" stage A lesions, stage A prostatic cancer is by definition a pathologic diagnosis. Stage A tumors are often termed occult, latent, or microscopic prostatic carcinoma because the tumor is found histologically and unexpectedly in tissue removed for presumed benign prostatic hypertrophy. Most often, the lesion is detected when a transurethral prostatectomy or open enucleation of the prostate is performed in a situation where the prostate gland is thought to be benign by digital palpation (Fig 4–1). The incidence of stage A prostatic cancer increases progressively with age.[1]

Overall, approximately 10% of patients undergoing prostatectomy for presumed benign prostatic hyperplasia are found to have evidence of carcinoma on histologic examination of the surgical specimen. Nevertheless, the incidence of stage A prostatic cancer at autopsy is almost twice the recognized clinical incidence of the disease after prostatectomy in patients of corresponding ages.[2] Several factors may account for the difference between clinical and autopsy recognition of microscopic prostatic cancer. First of all, most prostatic cancers are thought to arise in the peripheral portions of the prostate or in the prostatic capsule. It is for this reason that a simple prostatectomy, whether by the transurethral or open method, is not protective against the future development of prostatic cancer.[3] The thoroughness of the surgeon's resection of prostatic tissue as well as the pathologist's histologic examination may profoundly influence the incidence of the disease after prostatectomy. In the survey of the American College of Surgeons, 26% of patients overall with prostatic cancer had stage A disease at the time of diagnosis.[4]

SUBCLASSIFICATION OF STAGE A PROSTATIC CANCER

The marked difference between the incidence of prostatic cancer detected at autopsy and the clinical prevalence of the disease leads to the conclusion

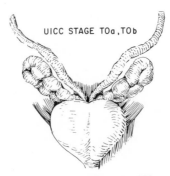

UICC STAGE TOa,TOb

STAGE A PROSTATE CANCER

FIG 4–1.
Digital palpation of the prostate is normal in patients with stage A carcinoma. No nodules or areas of induration suspicious for carcinoma should be evident.

that the natural history of most stage A prostatic cancers is one in which a prolonged time to disease progression occurs. Furthermore, the substantial majority of patients with low-grade stage A1 tumors never develop clinically evident disease. On the other hand, there are some patients with stage A disease, especially those with diffuse involvement or high-grade tumors, in whom clinically significant or metastatic tumor develops. Recognition of this difference led to subdivision of stage A tumors into A1 and A2 categories. Jewett[5] proposed this division in 1975 because of the accumulating evidence for significant difference in prognosis between focal and diffuse disease.

Stage A1

In general, stage A1 prostatic cancer implies low-volume and low-grade tumor. Unfortunately, there are no uniformly accepted criteria for definition of stage A1 prostatic cancer. Most classification systems agree that poorly differentiated tumors should not be categorized as stage A1 lesions regardless of the extent of disease. Other criteria used vary from determination of the number of foci of tumor, the number of prostatic chips involved after a transurethral prostatectomy, or assessment of the percentage involvement of the resected specimen. Often, involvement of fewer than three to five foci of disease or less than 5% of the total specimen is considered stage A1 disease.[6] At the University of Utah, patients are categorized as having stage A1 disease when there are five or fewer foci of tumor detected. Although this is inherently an arbitrary figure, it does seem to identify adequately patients who likely have clinically insignificant tumor. Tumor grade and extent are closely related, and their effects on prognosis are difficult to separate. Nearly 90% of well-differentiated tumors are associated with focal lesions, while 80% of less differentiated patterns are associated with diffuse involvement.[7]

Identification of stage A1 tumor generally implies that the disease is clinically insignificant and unlikely to progress within the lifetime of the patient. Several studies have shown cancer progression rates of less than 8% over a variable period of follow-up.[7, 8] Cantrell and associates[9] found tumor progression in only 2% of patients with stage A1 tumor who were followed for a minimum of four years. However, a follow-up report from the same institution showed that 16% of the patients had developed disease progression when they were at risk for eight years or longer.[10] In this series, stage A1 was defined as 5% or less tumor involvement of the entire specimen. Blute and associates[11] found disease progression a mean of ten years later in four (27%) of 15 patients aged 60 years or younger at the time of diagnosis of stage A1 disease.

Stage A2

Stage A2 prostatic cancer is thought to be more aggressive than stage A1 disease and more likely to be a competing cause of death or morbidity in an individual patient. Although most incidentally discovered prostatic cancers are classified as stage A1 disease, up to one third of patients have diffuse involvement or poorly differentiated tumors, i.e., stage A2.[12] Just as the criteria for definition of stage A1 tumors vary, there is no uniform agreement about what constitutes a stage A2 prostatic cancer. Generally, greater than five foci or more than 5% total involvement of the resected specimen is considered stage A2 disease as well as any poorly differentiated tumor regardless of the area of involvement.

Several studies have shown that the prognosis for stage A2 prostatic cancer patients is more ominous than that for Stage A1 disease.[13] Stage A2 tumors have a higher incidence of pelvic lymph node metastasis and involvement of the prostatic capsule.[14, 15] Heaney and associates[7] found that 28% of patients with stage A2 prostatic cancer had disease progression with no treatment or endocrine therapy alone. Fifteen percent of patients died of prostatic cancer with a variable period of follow-up, but most had been followed at least ten years. Cantrell and associates[9] found disease progression in 48% of their stage A2 prostatic cancer patients and cancer death in 22%.

DETERMINATION OF STAGE

Although the distinction between stage A1 and stage A2 prostatic cancer is arbitrary, this system of subclassification seems valid and important. Although generalizations may not be applicable in an individual situation, most patients with stage A1 prostatic cancer never develop clinically evident tumor, while those with stage A2 lesions have more significant disease that may affect their overall survival. Because of this, it is imperative that the classification of patients as having stage A1 or stage A2 disease be accurate.

By definition, all patients with stage A disease have a prostate that was felt to be benign by digital palpation preoperatively. Most often, tissue is removed by transurethral resection because of bladder outlet obstructive symptoms. Upon histologic examination of the resected tissue, the pathologist identifies one or more foci of adenocarcinoma.

Since transurethral resection of the prostate results in submission of many prostatic chips to the pathologist, a pertinent question is how many chips should be examined as a routine in order to detect stage A prostatic cancer. It is impractical to examine all chips in every patient undergoing prostatectomy, and most pathologists examine a "representative" number of chips. Murphy and associates[16] found that examination of 6 gm of tissue from a TURP specimen identified all patients with stage A2 disease.[16] Fewer than 10% of patients with carcinoma were not identified by this method, and all had stage A1 tumor. Therefore, routine examination of the entire submitted specimen is not necessary, and about 10 gm of the specimen should be examined. If any carcinoma is identified, all of the remaining chips should be submitted and representative sections taken so that the exact number of foci of tumor can be determined. If carcinoma is detected after open enucleation of a clinically benign prostate, multiple sections should be taken in order to determine the percent involvement of the gland.

PELVIC LYMPH NODE METASTASIS

The frequency with which pelvic lymph node metastasis occurs is a rough reflection of the metastatic potential for a given stage of prostatic cancer. Pelvic node dissection has been performed as part of a staging evaluation in 40 patients with stage A1 carcinoma of the prostate at the University of Utah. No patient was found to have histologic evidence of involvement of the pelvic lymph nodes. This finding lends credence to the clinical impression of the indolent nature of most stage A1 prostatic cancers and leads to the conclusion that pelvic node dissection is neither necessary nor justified in patients with stage A1 prostatic cancer. Similarly, pelvic lymphangiography, CT scanning, or MRI imaging of the pelvis add no useful information.

On the other hand, pelvic lymph node metastasis has been documented in approximately one fourth of patients with stage A2 disease undergoing pelvic node dissection. This rate exceeds the incidence of nodal metastasis in patients with stage B1 nodules and approaches that of stage B2 carcinoma. Thus, development of a palpable nodule is not required for prostatic cancer to realize its malignant and metastatic potential. Tumor grade can be a fairly accurate predictor of the status of the pelvic lymph nodes in patients with stage A2 tumors. No patient with a well-differentiated stage A2 lesion (Gleason score of 2–4) had positive nodes at pelvic lymphadenectomy compared with 26% of those with moderately differentiated cancer and 38% of those with a Gleason score of 8–10. Based upon these findings, pelvic lymph node evaluation, preferably by surgical node dissection, should be performed as part of staging in patients with stage A2 carcinoma who are being considered for definitive therapy, especially if the tumor is moderately or poorly differentiated.

THE ROLE OF REPEATED TRANSURETHRAL RESECTION

A frequent concern when stage A1 carcinoma is identified is that the transurethral resection or enucleation may have sampled only a small part of a diffusely infiltrating cancer that would more appropriately be classified as stage A2. The accuracy of separating patients with incidental carcinoma of the prostate into focal or diffuse categories depends upon how well the transurethral resection (TUR) or open prostatectomy specimen reflects the true extent of the tumor. The resection or enucleation may leave behind microscopic foci of cancer in some patients while removing all of the tumor in others. Since prostatic cancer is thought to arise in the peripheral portion of the gland, tumor found in the specimen may merely be the superficial portion of a deeper, more diffuse cancer. Understaging may result in failure to employ potentially curative therapy in patients with diffuse and more aggressive tumors.

Because of these concerns, repeated transurethral resection of the prostate has been used for further staging of A1 tumors. Usually, a period of approximately three months elapses between the initial resection and the repeat procedure. Since the initial resection should have removed all of the tissue to the level of the prostatic capsule, the repeat resection usually results in removal of only 5 to 10 gm of tissue. A special effort should be made to remove all of the posterior tissue since this is the area wherein most cancers arise. McMillen and Wettlaufer[17] reviewed their experience in a series of 27 stage A1 patients undergoing repeated TUR. They found residual tumor in 11 cases (37%) and reclassified these patients as stage A2.

Identification of *any* residual carcinoma on a repeated TUR should not necessarily result in upstaging of the patient to stage A2. The issue of what constitutes "significant" residual tumor should be considered. Patients should remain stage A1 if the amount of residual tumor on repeated TUR plus the amount of tumor on the original resection is within the criteria used to define stage A1 disease at the initial diagnosis. Such patients presumably have the same prognosis as is reported for stage A1 patients not undergoing repeated TUR. Therefore, patients should be considered to have "significant" residual tumor only if the total number of foci exceeds five. Most often, when repeat TUR is performed and residual carcinoma detected, only one or two foci of tumor are found and diffuse tumor is rarely identified.[18]

Experience at the University of Utah suggests that the intial TUR accurately reflects the true extent of cancer in the majority of patients. Of 55 patients classified as stage A1, only two (3.5%) had what was considered to be significant residual tumor on a repeat TUR. Eighty-two percent of patients had no tumor at all identified. An additional 14.5% of patients had focal residual tumor

TABLE 4–1.

Pathologic Findings on Repeat TUR or Radical Prostatectomy In Stage A1 Carcinoma

PROCEDURE (NO. OF PATIENTS)	NO RESIDUAL TUMOR, NO. (%)	RESIDUAL TUMOR, FOCAL, NO. (%)	RESIDUAL TUMOR, DIFFUSE, NO. (%)
Repeat TUR (55)	45 (82)	8 (14.5)	2 (3.5)
Radical prostatectomy (31)	16 (52)	11 (35)	4 (13)
Total (86)	**61** (71)	**19** (22)	**6** (7)

identified that did not result in reclassification as stage A2 since the volume of residual cancer was not considered clinically significant (Table 4–1).

The finding of residual tumor may imply that the original cancer was multicentric. Indeed, a significant number of incidental cancers of the prostate may be multicentric in origin. Edwards and associates[19] found this to be the case in 8 of 29 prostate glands with unsuspected carcinoma found at autopsy. The clinical signficance of this finding is unknown. Whitmore[20] suggests that patients with incidental carcinoma of the prostate that is multifocal may be expected to have a long survival without additional treatment. In the vast majority of reports on incidental prostatic cancer, stage A1 disease is defined according to the number of foci or percent involvement without regard to whether the tumor originates from a single or multicentric lesion. Furthermore, it is not possible to make this distinction clinically.

Although residual cancer may remain after a transurethral resection, it is important to distinguish focal from diffuse tumor. Only a distinct minority of patients are found to have diffuse residual carcinoma after a repeat transurethral resection. Therefore, it seems that the initial TUR itself is an adequate staging procedure in the majority of patients with stage A1 prostatic cancer. A repeat resection does not contribute significantly to staging accuracy.

TREATMENT OPTIONS

Radical Prostatectomy

Radical prostatectomy has been performed in some patients with stage A1 carcinoma. As would be anticipated, long-term survival rates are excellent. However, the prevailing sentiment is that such therapy is overly aggressive since the prognosis is good even in the absence of treatment in most patients.

Thirty-one patients at the University of Utah have undergone radical prostatectomy for stage A1 carcinoma. Fifty-two percent of patients had no residual tumor detected in the radical prostatectomy specimen. An additional 35% of patients had only focal residual tumor that probably was clinically insignificant. Only 13% of patients had diffuse residual tumor. Therefore, based upon pathologic findings alone, the substantial majority of patients underwent surgery that likely was unnecessary. A subset of patients with stage A1 disease and moderately differentiated histologic characteristics was also studied. In this group of

TABLE 4–2.

Findings on Repeat TUR or Radical Prostatectomy According to Tumor Grade on Original TUR in Stage A1

GLEASON SCORE (NO. OF PATIENTS)	NO RESIDUAL TUMOR, NO. (%)	RESIDUAL TUMOR FOCAL, NO. (%)	RESIDUAL TUMOR DIFFUSE, NO. (%)
2,3,4 (70)	53 (76)	15 (21)	2 (3)
5,6,7 (12)	7 (58)	3 (25)	2 (17)

TABLE 4–3.

Pathologic Findings on Radical Prostatectomy According to Extent of Tumor on TUR in Stage A1

NO. OF FOCI ON TUR (NO. OF PATIENTS)	NO RESIDUAL TUMOR, NO. (%)	RESIDUAL TUMOR FOCAL, NO. (%)	RESIDUAL TUMOR DIFFUSE, NO. (%)
1 to 3 (22)	11 (50)	9 (41)	2 (9)
4 or 5 (9)	5 (56)	2 (22)	2 (22)
Total	**16** (51.5)	**11** (35.5)	**4** (13)

patients, 58% had no residual tumor, 25% had focal residual carcinoma, and 17% had residual diffuse tumor. Although there was a higher incidence of diffuse residual tumor in these patients, the majority still had histologic findings that would not seem to justify the procedure (Table 4–2).

Examination of radical prostatectomy specimens based simply upon the number of foci of carcinoma detected on the TUR is only minimally helpful in identifying patients with diffuse residual tumor who may benefit from radical prostatectomy. If patients with only one to three foci of tumor are evaluated, half have no residual carcinoma, whereas 9% have diffuse residual tumor. Of those with four or five foci on the initial TUR, 56% have no residual tumor compared with 22% with diffuse residual carcinoma (Table 4–3).

Because of the inability to identify preoperatively the small percentage of patients who have apparently significant tumor based upon histologic findings, radical prostatectomy should not be recommended to patients with stage A1 carcinoma on a routine basis. In young patients (generally those younger than 65 years) with moderately differentiated histologic findings, radical prostatectomy may be justifiable.

Patients with stage A2 disease generally have a worse prognosis than those with stage A1 carcinoma but are a heterogeneous population. Prognosis in an individual patient is difficult to predict. Survival rates after radical prostatectomy for stage A2 carcinoma generally have been good, with cancer progression rates of around 10%.[21, 22] Forty patients at the University of Utah with stage

A2 prostatic cancer have undergone radical prostatectomy. Ninety-one percent of patients are alive at five years and free of any evidence of recurrent disease. Only two patients have developed tumor recurrence during the period of follow-up. Although these results are excellent, the relatively short follow-up must be considered as well as the fact that patients with positive lymph nodes were excluded from the group.

Despite the relatively limited clinical data and follow-up of patients with stage A2 prostatic cancer undergoing radical prostatectomy, the operation does appear to be justified in this patient group based upon the histologic findings. Seventy-four percent of patients are found to have diffuse residual carcinoma after radical prostatectomy, and 9% have no residual tumor in the surgical specimen.

In an attempt to differentiate further the patients with diffuse tumor from those with focal or no residual carcinoma, patients have been analyzed according to the grade of the initial lesion. Although 27% of patients with well-differentiated Gleason patterns had no residual carcinoma, nearly half (46%) had diffuse disease compared to 88% of those with poorly differentiated lesions (Table 4–4). Extent of disease (number of foci) also correlates to some degree with pathologic findings. Patients with a "small" A2 lesion on transurethral resection were considered. This category was defined as 6 to 17 foci of carcinoma in the transurethral specimen (3% to 15% total involvement). In this group, 42% of patients had diffuse residual carcinoma after radical prostatectomy and one had histologic extension to the seminal vesicle.

These pathologic findings show that stage A2 prostatic cancer is indeed a heterogeneous population. Although there is a subgroup of patients with A2 disease who may not benefit from aggressive therapy, neither histologic grade nor extent of tumor on transurethral resection reliably identifies these patients. There is some correlation between these factors and subsequent pathologic findings, but their predictive value in an individual case is limited. Based upon pathologic data and survival rates as well as the assumption that significant histologic residual disease implies clinically significant cancer, staging pelvic lymph node dissection and radical prostatectomy seem both justifiable and a reasonable therapeutic approach for patients with stage A2 prostatic cancer and a 10- to 15-year life expectancy.

TABLE 4–4.

Pathologic Findings From Radical Prostatectomy and Pelvic Lymphadenectomy According to Grade in Patients With Stage A2 Carcinoma

NO. OF PATIENTS	GLEASON SCORE	RESIDUAL TUMOR			
		NONE, NO. (%)	FOCAL, NO. (%)	DIFFUSE, NO. (%)	POS. NODES, NO. (%)
11	2–4	3 (27)	3 (27)	5 (46)	0
15	5–7	0	2 (13.5)	11 (73)	2 (13.5)
8	8–10	0	1 (12.5)	7 (88)	6 (75)

In some patients, radical prostatectomy may be more difficult after a previous TURP. Tissue planes may be somewhat obliterated, and periprostatic scarring can occur. Nichols and associates[21] believed that complications were fewer and the operation was easier if patients underwent radical prostatectomy within six weeks of the TURP. Others have recommended waiting at least three months after TUR before performing radical surgery. We have found that the interval between the TURP and radical prostatectomy is not of critical importance and the complication rate in stage A2 patients is not significantly different from that seen in other stages of the disease.

External Radiation

Just as radical prostatectomy is unnecessary in most patients with stage A1 prostatic cancer, external irradiation is not indicated. However, external beam therapy is an option in patients with stage A2 prostatic cancer who have a life expectancy of 10 to 15 years. Most commonly, four-field rotational treatment is used with 10×10-cm portals and a total prostatic dose of 6,500 to 7,000 rad. In general, at least six weeks should elapse between the prostatectomy and the initiation of irradiation so that some reepithelization of the prostatic fossa can occur.

Lymph node evaluation should be performed prior to external irradiation. If the nodes are positive, treatment is unlikely to impart any survival benefit. Approximately one fourth of patients with stage A2 prostatic cancer are found to have histologic evidence of pelvic node metastasis after a pelvic lymphadenectomy. Detection of pelvic node metastases by other methods such as CT scanning or lymphangiography occurs in only around 10% of patients with stage A2 carcinoma. Therefore, if accurate staging is to occur, a lymph node dissection should be performed prior to radiation.

Unfortunately, only very limited data are available regarding the efficacy of external irradiation in patients with stage A2 prostatic cancer. In most series, stage A and B lesions have not been segregated. Bagshaw's series include stage A cancers under the category of "disease limited to the prostate," which also includes all stage B cancers.[23] McGowan[24] reported a 97% five-year survival in patients with stage A carcinoma treated by external beam irradiation. However, the series included patients with stage A1 tumors, and follow-up of only five years is insufficient to allow any comment regarding treatment efficacy.

Interstitial Irradiation

Interstitial implantation of iodine 125 seeds has been unsatisfactory in patients with stage A prostatic cancer. Implantation of 40 to 50 seeds often is necessary to achieve optimal dosimetry. After a thorough prostatectomy, there frequently is insufficient residual tissue to support implantation of this number of seeds.

When Au 198 isotopes are used, only six to ten seeds are implanted in the prostate and a boost of external irradiation is used. Therefore, the technique is feasible even after prostatectomy. In the Baylor University series, 67% of patients with stage A2 prostatic cancer were alive at 10 years and 46% were without evidence of disease.[25] The results do not seem to be significantly different from those seen in stage A2 patients not receiving any treatment to the primary tumor.

Iridium 192 has been used in some patients with stage A prostatic cancer. Clinical experience is quite limited and survival figures are not available.[26]

SUMMARY

Approximately 10% of patients undergoing prostatectomy for presumed BPH are found to have microscopic evidence of carcinoma. The majority of these patients have only occasional foci of well-differentiated cancer that is considered to be stage A1 disease. Prognosis in these patients generally is excellent, and prostatic cancer rarely is a competing cause of death or significant morbidity. Overall rates of cancer progression are around 7% although cancer progression has been seen in up to 25% of young patients followed for long periods of time. Therefore, treatment of stage A1 carcinoma is not indicated, except perhaps in young patients (generally younger than 60 to 65 years).

Repeat transurethral prostatectomy has been of limited benefit in identifying the small percentage of patients with stage A1 carcinoma who harbor diffuse tumor in the residual prostatic tissue. After a repeat TUR, either no tumor or occasional foci of carcinoma is usually detected, and this often does not influence the therapeutic decision. Therefore, if a complete removal of the obstructive prostatic tissue has been performed, the histologic findings on the initial resection are usually indicative of the overall tumor status.

Stage A2 prostatic cancer involves more extensive portions of the gland, generally more than five foci or greater than 5% total involvement. Often, stage A2 cancers are of a higher grade than stage A1 lesions. Cancer progression rates and deaths from prostatic cancer are significant in patients with stage A2 tumors. Approximately 25% of patients are found to have histologic evidence of pelvic node metastasis. Thus, aggressive therapy with curative intent is justified in patients with a reasonable life expectancy (10 to 15 years).

Because of the relatively high incidence of nodal metastasis, lymph node evaluation should be performed. In general, lymph node staging should be by surgical pelvic lymphadenectomy. If the lymph nodes are normal histologically, definitive therapy should be employed. No strong recommendations for the type of therapy can be made based upon the limited data regarding long-term survival. However, radical prostatectomy has been well tolerated in this group of patients, with complication rates that probably do not exceed those seen in other stages of the disease. Most often, residual carcinoma is identified in the surgical specimen, but extracapsular extension or seminal vesicle invasion are relatively unusual. Therefore, in patients with histologically negative lymph nodes, radical prostatectomy accomplishes the goal of surgical removal of all known tumor. Ten-year survival rates in the limited series that are available approach those expected in a control group without prostatic cancer.

External irradiation has also been used to treat stage A2 prostatic cancer. Radiation portals should encompass the entire prostate and periprostatic region (approximately 10×10-cm fields). Analysis of survival data is difficult since most reported series have not segregated stage A patients from those with other stages of the disease. Experience with interstitial irradiation with Au 198 or Ir 192 is quite limited. Patients with stage A tumors are poorly selected for interstitial irradiation with iodine 125 since the remaining prostatic tissue frequently is insufficient to support the number of seeds needed for adequate dosimetry.

Because of the marked difference in prognosis between most patients with stage A1 carcinoma and those with more diffuse disease, treatment recommendations vary between the two subcategories of stage A disease. The clinical rate of tumor progression within the lifetime of the patient is low enough in the substantial majority of those with stage A1 lesions that no treatment generally is the most appropriate course. On the other hand, detection of stage A2 disease is a more significant finding, and some form of definitive therapy should be recommended in patients who otherwise have a life expectancy of at least 10 to 15 years.

REFERENCES

1. Whitmore WF Jr: The natural history of prostatic cancer. *Cancer* 1973; 32:1104–1112.
2. Denton SE, Choy SH, Valk WL: Occult prostatic carcinoma diagnosed by the step section technique of the surgical specimen. *J Urol* 1965; 93:296–298.
3. Smith GG, Woodruff LM: The development of cancer of the prostate after subtotal prostatectomy. *J Urol* 1950; 63:1077–1080.
4. Murphy GP, Natarajan N, Pontes JE, et al: The National Survey of Prostate Cancer in the United States by the American College of Surgeons. *J Urol* 1982; 127:928–934.
5. Jewett HJ: The present status of radical prostatectomy for stages A and B prostatic cancer. *Urol Clin North Am* 1975; 2:105.
6. Sheldon CA, Williams RD, Fraley EE: Incidental carcinoma of the prostate: A review of the literature and critical reappraisal of classification. *J Urol* 1980; 124:626.
7. Heaney JA, Chang HC, Daoy JJ, et al: Prognosis of clinically undiagnosed prostatic carcinoma and the influence of endocrine therapy. *J Urol* 1977; 118:283.
8. Correa RJ Jr, Anderson RG, Gibbons RP, et al: Latent carcinoma of the prostate— Why the controversy? *J Urol* 1974; 111:644–646.
9. Cantrell BB, DeKlerk DP, Eggleston JC, et al: Pathologic factors that influence prognosis in stage A prostatic cancer: The influence of extent versus grade. *J Urol* 1981; 125:516–520.
10. Epstein JI, Walsh PC, Eggleston JC: Prognosis of untreated stage A1 prostate carcinoma: A study of 94 cases with extended follow-up. *J Urol* 1986; 135:242–A.
11. Blute ML, Zincke H, Farrow GM: Long-term follow-up of young patients with stage A adenocarcinoma of the prostate. *J Urol* 1986; 136:840–843.

12. Golimbu M, Schinella R, Morales P, et al: Differences in pathologic characteristics and prognosis of clinical A2 prostatic cancer from A1 and B disease. *J Urol* 1978; 119:618.
13. Hanash KA, Utz DC, Cook EN: Carcinoma of the prostate: A 15-year follow-up. *J Urol* 1972; 107:450–453.
14. Parfitt HE Jr, Smith JA Jr, Seaman JP, et al: Surgical treatment of stage A2 prostatic carcinoma: Significance of tumor grade and extent. *J Urol* 1983; 129:763–765.
15. McNeal JE: Origin and development of carcinoma of the prostate. *Cancer* 1969; 23:24–34.
16. Murphy WM, Dean PJ, Brasfield JA, et al: Incidental carcinoma of the prostate: How much sampling is adequate? *Am J Surg Pathol* 1986; 10:170.
17. McMillen J, Wettlaufer JN: The role of repeat transurethral biopsy in stage A carcinoma of the prostate. *J Urol* 1976; 116:759.
18. Parfitt HE Jr, Smith JA Jr, Gliedman JB, et al: Accuracy of staging in A1 carcinoma of the prostate. *Cancer* 1983; 51:2346–2350.
19. Edwards CN, Steinthrosson E, Nicholson D: An autopsy study of latent prostatic cancer. *Cancer* 1953; 6:531.
20. Whitmore WF Jr: The natural history of prostatic cancer. *Cancer* 1973; 32:1104.
21. Nichols RT, Barry JM, Hodges CV: The morbidity of radical prostatectomy for multifocal stage 1 prostatic adenocarcinoma. *J Urol* 1977; 117:83–84.
22. Bass RB Jr, Barrett DM: Radical retropubic prostatectomy after transurethral resection. *J Urol* 1980; 124:495–497.
23. Bagshaw MA, Ray GR, Cox RS: Radiotherapy of prostatic carcinoma: Long- or short-term efficacy. *Urology* 1985; 25:17–23.
24. McGowan DG: Radiation therapy in the management of localized carcinoma of the prostate: A preliminary report. *Cancer* 1977; 39:98–102.
25. Scardino PT, Guerriero WG, Carlton CE Jr: Surgical staging and combined therapy with radioactive gold grain implantation and external irradiation, in Johnson DE, Boileau MA (eds): *Genitourinary Tumors: Fundamental Principles and Surgical Techniques.* New York, Grune & Stratton, 1982, p 85.
26. Court B, Tassagne D: Interstitial radiation therapy of cancer of the prostate using iridium 192 wires. *Cancer Treat Rep* 1977; 61:329–330.

5

Stage B Prostate Cancer

Few areas in urologic surgery have generated more controversy and disagreement among clinicians than the appropriate management of patients with stage B prostatic cancer. Although numerous retrospective series can be used to support a particular treatment bias, variations in staging techniques and patient selection invalidate many comparative attempts. Few randomized data exist, and studies with control groups of patients are sparse. Moreover, the prolonged natural history of the disease in some patients creates difficulty in determining the impact of treatment.

Because of these factors, dogmatic therapeutic recommendations in patients with stage B prostatic cancer frequently are unfounded. Therefore, it is incumbent upon the clinician to understand the relative risk imposed by a diagnosis of stage B prostatic cancer as well as the potential impact of treatment. Only in this manner can patients most likely to benefit from definitive therapy be selected while those with tumors unlikely to affect their survival can be spared the morbidity of some treatments.

DEFINITION

The category of stage B includes all patients with palpable tumors that are confined within the capsule of the prostate gland. In the American College of Surgeons survey, 29% of patients with prostatic cancer were found to have stage B lesions at the time of initial presentation.[1] Stage B prostatic cancer is almost always asymptomatic, and the palpable abnormality is usually detected on a routine physical examination. By definition, there is no evidence of distant metastatic spread, and symptoms of bladder outlet obstruction usually are due to concomitant benign prostatic hypertrophy rather than the carcinomatous component. The diagnosis is confirmed by a needle biopsy or aspiration of the prostate.

Stage B prostatic cancer is divided into two substages, B1 and B2. The distinction between stage B1 and B2 prostatic cancer is based upon the size and location of the palpable abnormality and is variably defined. The classic

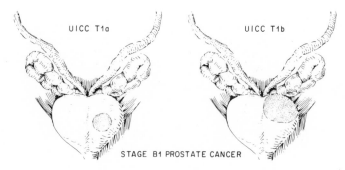

FIG 5–1.
State B1 adenocarcinoma of the prostate. A classic Jewett nodule *(left)* is less than 1½ cm in size and surrounded by normal-feeling prostatic tissue. In general, palpable nodules less than 2 cm in size that appear to be confined within the capsule of the prostate are considered to be stage B1 tumors *(right).*

"Jewett nodule" consists of a 1-cm distinct nodule surrounded by palpably normal prostatic tissue[2] (Fig 5–1). More broadly, B1 is defined as tumors that involve less than one lobe of the prostate. Patients at the University of Utah are categorized as having B1 nodules if the palpable intraprostatic nodule is 2 cm or less in diameter. Patients with lesions greater than 2 cm in diameter or two distinct tumor nodules are considered to have stage B2 disease (Fig 5–2).

Subclassification of patients into stage B1 and stage B2 disease is a reflection only of the volume of palpable tumor. Byar and Mostofi[3] found an 85% incidence of multifocal involvement of the prostate even in patients with apparently localized lesions. Whether this is related to multicentric origin of the

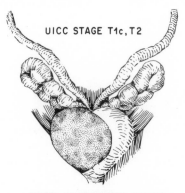

STAGE B2 PROSTATE CANCER

FIG 5–2.
Stage B2 adenocarcinoma includes tumors greater than 2 cm in size that are confined within the prostatic capsule. In addition, tumors in which there are two distinct nodules are considered to be stage B2 even if neither is larger than 1½ to 2 cm in size.

tumor or intragland metastasis is uncertain, but it does demonstrate that the palpable abnormality of the prostate often does not reflect the true extent of the disease.

NATURAL HISTORY OF STAGE B PROSTATIC CANCER

Determination of the natural history of stage B prostatic cancer is of critical importance in analyzing treatment results as well as in making therapeutic recommendations to patients. Unfortunately, the natural history of stage B prostatic cancer is poorly understood. An indolent, prolonged clinical course can be anticipated in some patients, while others are destined to develop rapid disease progression and death from prostatic cancer. Distinction between these groups is often not possible or, at best, inexact.

Hanash and associates[4] reported a five-year survival rate of only 19% in patients with stage B prostatic cancer treated conservatively. Treatment consisted solely of transurethral prostatectomy, and the substantial majority of patients had stage B2 lesions.

Other series have shown a lower incidence of disease progression and implied a generally more favorable natural history for most stage B prostatic tumors. The Veterans Administration Cooperative Urologic Research Group randomized patients with stage B prostatic cancer to placebo or placebo plus radical prostatectomy. The staging procedures used in this study were antiquated by modern standards and did not include bone scanning or pelvic lymph node assessment. Moreover, the numbers of patients involved were insufficient for valid statistical analysis. Nevertheless, with a median follow-up of 7.7 years, no definitive advantage for the radical prostatectomy group could be demonstrated. While the deficiencies of the study do not allow the conclusion that radical prostatectomy is ineffective or unnecessary treatment for stage B prostatic cancer, these results do lend credence to the concept that short-term survival may be good in many patients with stage B prostatic cancer even in the absence of effective therapy.

Whitmore[6] has followed 45 patients with clinical stage B prostatic cancer without treatment for a minimum of at least two years after histologic diagnosis. Fifteen patients showed evidence of disease progression a mean of 59 months after diagnosis. The remaining 30 patients have been followed a mean of 79 months without clinically apparent progression in stage. This experience can be used to verify both the relatively indolent nature of some stage B prostatic cancers as well as the rapid disease progression that can be observed in others. Overall, though, the demonstration that disease progression (often to stage D) was observed in one third of the patients with a relatively short mean follow-up (six years) suggests that stage B prostatic cancer represents a serious threat to patients who otherwise have a life expectancy of at least 10 to 15 years. The implication, however, that therapeutic intervention by whatever means could favorably influence these results does not necessarily follow. Cautious, yet pertinent, interpretation would allow the suggestion that the patients demonstrating disease progression in these series of untreated patients are those less likely to respond favorably to therapy, while those whose tumors have a more prolonged natural history are the ones likely to have a good result after treatment.

Further evidence of the aggressive nature of at least some stage B prostatic cancers is the demonstration that histologic pelvic lymph node metastasis is demonstrable in a significant number of patients, especially those with higher grade tumors. Approximately one third of patients with stage B1 prostatic cancer have well-differentiated lesions histologically, and pelvic lymph node metastasis has been demonstrated in only 4% of these patients. Moderately differentiated tumors are seen in the majority of patients with B1 lesions (60%) and nodal metastasis is evident in 14% of this group. Poorly differentiated histologic findings are uncommon in clinical stage B1 tumors, but up to one third of this group can be expected to have lymph node metastasis. Overall, pelvic node disease has been found in 12% of patients with stage B1 carcinoma of the prostate.[7]

Typically, there is a trend toward less differentiated histologic findings in stage B2 prostatic cancer and a corresponding increased incidence of pelvic nodal disease.[7] Only 18% of patients with stage B2 prostatic cancer are found to have well-differentiated lesions; 69% have moderately differentiated cancer, and 13% have poorly differentiated histologic findings. Pelvic lymph node metastasis is demonstrated in 18%, 27%, and 43% of patients, respectively. Overall, close to one third of patients with clinical stage B2 prostatic cancer have histologic evidence of pelvic lymph node metastasis demonstrable after pelvic lymphadenectomy (Table 5–1).

TREATMENT OPTIONS

One of the most difficult and important decisions for the clinician seeing patients with prostatic cancer is whether or not to recommend *any* treatment to a patient with a stage B prostatic tumor. The basis of clinical judgment is to compare the risk of the disease versus the impact of treatment and the life

TABLE 5–1.
Incidence of Pelvic Node Metastasis in Stage B Prostatic Cancer

	GRADE			
STAGE	WELL DIFFERENTIATED	MODERATELY DIFFERENTIATED	POORLY DIFFERENTIATED	TOTAL
B1	2/53 (4%)	13/94 (14%)	3/9 (33%)	**18/156** (12%)
B2	5/27 (18%)	29/106 (27%)	9/27 (43%)	**43/154** (28%)

expectancy of the patient. Strict age criteria as a basis for treatment recommendations are inappropriate since other factors may have a greater impact upon expected longevity than chronological age. However, most clinicians would agree that a diagnosis of stage B prostatic cancer in an otherwise healthy man 65 years of age or younger implies a significant threat and that aggressive therapy is warranted. On the other hand, most patients older than 75 years with stage B tumors are likely to die of competing causes before symptomatic progression of prostatic cancer that cannot be controlled by conservative measures is evident.

Unfortunately, the age at which stage B prostatic cancer is diagnosed often falls between these extremes. Numerous factors must be considered in determining the potential longevity of a patient and, thereby, the relative threat prostatic cancer poses. However, efforts at definitive management of stage B prostatic cancer are warranted in patients who otherwise have a reasonable life expectancy of 10 to 15 years. Although curative efforts may be justified in some patients, definitive demonstration of a favorable influence upon survival from any treatment method is difficult. Nevertheless, a commonly held and reasonably supported conclusion is that several methods of treatment have offered longer survival free of disease than would be expected in untreated patients. Categorical recommendation of one treatment method over another is not justifiable based upon the available data. However, extensive experience in uncontrolled series of prostatic cancer patients has been accumulated, and a number of observations are pertinent and valid.

Radical Prostatectomy

Radical prostatectomy for treatment of stage B prostatic cancer was reported by Young in 1905.[8] Since the natural history of untreated stage B prostatic cancer generally is prolonged, it has been thought that 15-year follow-up is necessary to assess the impact of treatment. Few series are available with patient follow-up of this duration. Furthermore, follow-up periods this long exclude from analysis patients who have been staged by modern criteria, including bone scan and pelvic lymph node dissection. However, Jewett[9] reported results in 103 patients undergoing radical perineal prostatectomy before 1951. All patients had B1 nodules, and the estimated survival at 15 years was 27%. Thirty-seven percent of patients died of prostatic cancer, but nearly half of these had microscopic invasion of the seminal vesicles. Jewett also performed radical prostatectomy in 79 patients with stage B2 tumors. Fifteen-year tumor-free survival was only 18%, but 50% of the patients had histologic invasion of the seminal vesicles.[9] In a later series of 57 patients from The Johns Hopkins Hospital undergoing radical prostatectomy for stage B1 disease, 15-year estimated tumor-free survival was 51%, a figure quite close to the expected survival of a general population of comparable age.[10] (Table 5–2).

Other series have shown relatively good long-term survival in patients with stage B prostatic cancer treated by radical prostatectomy. Hodges et al.[11] re-

TABLE 5–2.

Results of Radical Prostatectomy for Stage B Prostatic Cancer

| | | | SURVIVAL | |
	AUTHOR	NO. OF PATIENTS	5 YR	15 YR
Stage B1				
	Jewett	103	76%	27%
	Walsh & Jewett	57		51% (estimated)
	Hodges	195 (includes some stage A)	80%	27%
	Gibbons et al.	26	95%	54%
	Middleton & Smith	48	91%	(disease free)
Stage B2				
	Jewett	79	60%	18% (50% of patients had microscopic seminal vesicle invasion)
	Middleton & Smith	65	81% (disease free)	

ported a 15-year disease-free survival of 27% in a combined series. Gibbons and associates followed 26 patients with stage B1 for a minimum of 15 years and observed a survival rate of 54% (14 patients).

Numerous reports of excellent five-year survival after radical prostatectomy for stage B prostatic cancer have emerged. At the University of Utah, 44 patients with stage B1 prostatic cancer have undergone radical prostatectomy and been followed for five years.[12] Forty patients (91%) were alive and free of disease at five years. Of 58 patients with stage B2 tumors followed for at least five years, 47 (81%) were alive without evidence of disease.[13] It should be emphasized that five-year follow-up is clearly insufficient in patients with stage B prostatic cancer and that these survival figures are preliminary. Substantially fewer patients have been followed for ten years. However, death from prostatic cancer increased significantly between six and ten years. Three of the six patients with stage B1 tumors followed for at least 10 years had died of their disease. Twenty-seven patients with stage B2 tumors had been followed for ten years. Only seven patients were alive and free of disease.

Only two randomized studies of radical prostatectomy for stage B disease have been conducted. In the VACURG study, patients were randomized to radical prostatectomy plus placebo or placebo alone. No survival advantage for radical prostatectomy could be demonstrated; however, patient numbers were small, follow-up was limited, and there was an unequal distribution of tumor grade within the groups. Significantly more patients in the radical prostatectomy group had higher-grade tumors.

The Uro-Oncology Research Group conducted a prospective trial wherein patients with stage A or B prostatic cancer were randomized to radical prostatectomy or external irradiation.[14] Staging was similar in both groups and included serum acid phosphatase evaluation, bone scan, and pelvic lymphadenectomy. Time to first treatment failure was the study end point, and a positive prostate biopsy alone was not considered treatment failure in the radiation group. At the time of the report, treatment failure had occurred in 40% of the patients in the radiation therapy arm compared with only 10% of patients treated by radical prostatectomy. These results were statistically significant ($P < .05$). Thus, despite the difficulties in analyzing the various data, radical prostatectomy has endured as a treatment capable of providing long-term disease-free survival rates in patients with stage B prostatic cancer that appear to exceed those seen after other forms of therapy or observation alone.

Management of Patients With Microscopic Extracapsular Extension

A consistent observation is that patients with histologic evidence of microscopic tumor extension beyond the prostatic capsule, especially to the seminal vesicles, have a prognosis significantly poorer than that of patients whose disease is confined within the prostatic capsule. In the Johns Hopkins series, only 5% of patients with seminal vesicle involvement lived 15 years. Even with short-term follow-up, seminal vesicle invasion can be shown to be a poor prognostic parameter (Fig 5–3). In the Utah series, 50% of patients with microscopic seminal vesicle invasion had evidence of tumor recurrence within five

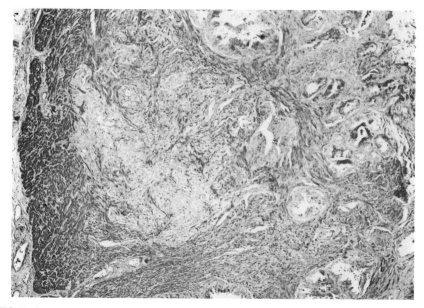

FIG 5–3.
Microscopic seminal vesicle invasion detected in a patient undergoing radical prostatectomy for a presumed stage B2 adenocarcinoma. Seminal vesicle invasion is a poor prognostic finding.

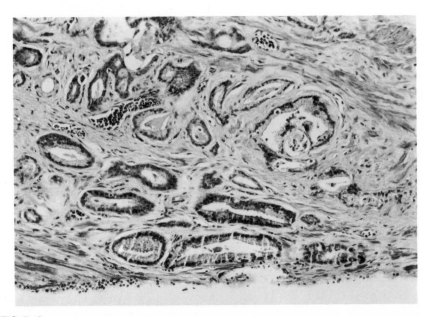

FIG 5–4.
Invasion of the prostatic capsule by adenocarcinoma identified after a radical prostatectomy. Capsular invasion alone has not had an adverse influence on local recurrence rates or overall patient survival.

years. Of apparently less concern is capsular penetration if surgical margins are otherwise adequate (Fig 5–4).

Since only a distinct minority of patients with seminal vesicle invasion fare well after radical prostatectomy alone, efforts should be made to identify patients with seminal vesicle involvement and exclude them from radical surgery. Elder et al.[15] found that 17% of their patients with apparent stage B1 nodules had microscopic seminal vesicle invasion and over 50% of patients with stage B2 cancers had histologic involvement of the seminal vesicles. However, preoperative staging in these patients was based primarily on digital palpation of the prostate. In particular, no method of assessment of the pelvic lymph nodes was performed.

Patients at the University of Utah with stage B2 prostatic cancer have been carefully evaluated regarding the postoperative histologic findings. Fifty patients with clinical stage B2 tumors and histologically negative lymph nodes underwent radical prostatectomy. Only two patients (4%) were found to have seminal vesicle involvement.[16] Catalona et al.[17] reported similar results. Careful digital palpation of the prostate combined with pelvic lymphadenectomy has improved the clinical staging of patients with stage B prostatic cancer and allowed exclusion of most patients with seminal vesicle invasion from radical surgery. The ability of transrectal ultrasonography to detect nonpalpable seminal vesicle invasion has not been tested adequately.

Despite this, unanticipated histologic extracapsular tumor extension and seminal vesicle involvement are seen in some patients after radical prostatectomy performed for presumed stage B disease. Strictly defined, these patients have pathologic stage C disease. Postoperative external beam irradiation has been used as a potential means to decrease local recurrence and improve survival in this group of patients. Lange and Narayan[18] were able to show that postoperative irradiation was reasonably well tolerated and that the incidence of incontinence and anastomotic stricture did not appear to be increased in their patients. However, Gibbons[19] found that postoperative radiotherapy increased the incidence of vesicourethral stricture and complications in his patients.

The ability of postoperative irradiation to improve long-term survival has not been demonstrated, although the incidence of local recurrence appears to be decreased. Ray and associates[20] found improved survival in patients undergoing external beam irradiation immediately after surgery compared with those treated when local recurrence was evident. However, these clearly are not comparable patient groups. Twenty-five patients with histologic extracapsular extension after radical prostatectomy at the University of Utah have been treated with postoperative irradiation ranging from 5,400 to 7,000 rad.[21] These patients have been compared retrospectively to a similar group of patients not treated with irradiation. Hormonal therapy was not employed in either group unless there was evidence of disease progression. No local recurrences were observed in the irradiated patients, while seven patients (17%) of those not receiving irradiation developed palpable local recurrence. Disease-free survival was similar in both groups, with distant disease being the most common cause of treatment failure in both groups.

None of these studies allows definitive conclusions regarding the role of radiation as a postoperative adjunct to radical prostatectomy. Although the treatment is relatively well tolerated, a somewhat increased rate of complications can be expected. The incidence of local recurrence seems to be decreased, but no favorable impact upon survival can be demonstrated. Considering this, the most prudent general recommendation seems to be that postoperative radiation should not be used as a routine or in patients with capsular penetration only. Patients with seminal vesicle involvement are at high risk for both local and distant failure and may be benefited by postoperative irradiation.

External Irradiation

In the 1970s, external irradiation emerged as an alternative to radical prostatectomy as a treatment method for stage B prostatic cancer. Initially, the ability to avoid the necessity for a surgical procedure as well as elimination of some of the complications of radical prostatectomy increased the attraction of external irradiation. Five-year survival and local control rates in stage B patients were excellent. Although external irradiation remains an alternative that should be considered in stage B prostatic cancer, several factors need to be examined more closely.

In most early series of prostatic cancer patients and in many current ones, lymph node evaluation has not been performed. Whole-pelvis treatment portals were employed based on the feeling that treatment should be delivered whether lymph nodes contained metastatic tumor or not. Since external beam irradiation has been shown to be incapable of prolonging survival in patients with positive pelvic nodes, most clinicians would agree that pelvic lymph node assessment should be performed prior to irradiation. Patients with positive nodes should be excluded from the morbidity and expense of such therapy. In most patients with stage B prostatic cancer, CT scanning or lymphangiography fail to detect pelvic lymph node involvement since lymph node metastases frequently are microscopic. Therefore, staging by pelvic lymph node dissection may be useful prior to external irradiation. If subsequent radiation portals are limited to the prostate and periprostatic region, treatment morbidity is not increased by the combined approach of surgery and irradiation.

Just as the morbidity of radical prostatectomy has been decreased in recent years, technical advances have lowered the complication rate after radiation treatment. In addition, limiting the radiation portals to the prostate and periprostatic region decreases the incidence of acute and chronic radiation cystitis or enteritis. Approximately 50% of patients who are sexually active before radiation become impotent after treatment, a figure similar to that obtained by most surgeons using the potency-sparing technique for radical prostatectomy.

The results of radiation therapy for prostatic cancer are difficult to assess. Most patients have not been subjected to lymph node dissection. Since approximately 15% of patients with stage B1 tumors are found to have lymph node metastasis, and up to one third of those with stage B2 lesions have nodal disease, failure to perform lymph node assessment creates a bias against radiation in reviewing results since most series include some patients with undetected stage D1 disease. In addition, stage A and B prostatic cancer frequently are included in the category of "disease limited to the prostate." The known differences in the natural history and treatment responsiveness of stage A and B prostatic cancer make analysis of patients grouped in this fashion extremely difficult. Finally, the relatively recent use of radiation therapy as definitive treatment of prostatic cancer limits the number of patients who have been followed for extended periods of time.

Bagshaw and colleagues[22] have reported the largest and most extensively followed group of patients treated with external irradiation for prostatic cancer. Patients were categorized as having disease limited to the prostate (stage A plus stage B) or extracapsular extension. The actuarial survival rate was 80% at 5 years, 58% at 10 years, and 37% at 15 years.[23] Although these figures are based upon actuarial survival and do include patients with stage A disease, long-term survival after radiation treatment for stage B prostatic cancer is demonstrable in selected patients.

Pilepich and associates[24] reported a five-year disease-free survival of 80% in patients with stage B prostatic cancer. McGowan[25] reported a five-year disease-free survival of 70% in patients with stage B1 tumors but only 38% in those with stage B2 lesions.

Analysis of retrospective series of patients with prostatic cancer treated by radiation is inexact for the reasons listed previously. The only randomized prospective study comparing external irradiation and radical prostatectomy, that conducted by the Uro-oncology Research Group, showed a statistically significant improvement in the time to first evidence of disease failure for patients undergoing radical prostatectomy.[14] Although this study should not be considered conclusive since further patient follow-up is necessary and corroborating studies should be performed, it does suggest the overall superiority of radical prostatectomy.

Postirradiation Biopsy

Although excellent short-term survival rates have been reported after external irradiation and good long-term actuarial survival in some series, concerns have been expressed regarding the high incidence of positive postirradiation biopsies in prostatic cancer patients. In Bagshaw's experience, 50% of patients with stage B prostatic cancer have had a positive biopsy result 18 or more months following irradiation.[25] Cox and Kline[26] reported a decreasing incidence of positive biopsy results as the interval between irradiation and biopsy increased. Furthermore, they believed that many of the positive biopsies contain cells that were "nonviable" and that serial biopsies did not predict local recurrence, distant metastasis, or probability of survival.[26]

Other studies have shown a direct correlation between postirradiation biopsy and patient survival.[27] Clearly, palpable prostatic regression and the conversion of biopsy findings from positive to negative may be somewhat delayed after external irradiation. However, a positive biopsy result 18 or more months after the completion of external irradiation is a poor prognostic finding and should be considered evidence of treatment failure.

It is difficult to generalize regarding appropriate treatment of patients with positive biopsy results after irradiation. Often, tumor progression may have occurred in the interval since completion of irradiation, and the radiation treatment itself may obscure some of the palpable tissue planes. Therefore, determination of the local extent of the actual tumor is inexact. However, if the palpable induration seems to be confined within the prostatic capsule, salvage radical prostatectomy after external irradiation is feasible and has a complication rate only minimally greater than that seen in nonirradiated patients. if there is evidence of tumor extension beyond the prostatic capsule, radical prostatectomy is inappropriate and hormonal therapy should be used when symptomatic disease progression becomes evident.

Interstitial Irradiation

Iodine 125

Interstitial implantation of iodine 125 seeds for treatment of prostatic cancer was initiated at Memorial Sloan-Kettering Cancer Center in the early

1970s.[26] Although the procedure has been associated with a low morbidity rate and has the advantage that erectile potency is preserved in more than 90% of patients, overall disease-free survival has been relatively disappointing in patients followed for sufficient periods of time. Tumor-free survival at five years was 66% for clinical stage B1 tumors and 30% for stage B2. However, it should be noted that these results are based upon clinical staging. Nearly half of the patients did not have bone scans, and one fourth had elevated serum acid phosphatase levels. If pathologic stage alone is considered, five-year survival rates for stage B tumors more closely approximate those obtained with alternative treatment methods.[27]

Palpable regression of tumors after iodine 125 implantation is slower than after external irradiation. In some patients, complete regression by palpation is not evident until three years after surgery. Schellhammer and associates[28] found positive biopsy specimens in 33% of patients between 12 and 18 months after iodine 125 implantation of the prostate, but in only 13% after 36 months. Thus, biopsies after iodine 125 implantation of the prostate may not be meaningful until at least three years after surgery.

The data suggesting that tumor-free survival after iodine 125 implantation for stage B prostatic cancer may be somewhat less than after radical prostatectomy are important, and the relatively high incidence of positive post-treatment biopsies is concerning. However, further data with long-term follow-up are necessary before definitive conclusions regarding the efficacy of this procedure are made. The procedure is of low morbidity with a relatively short hospitalization and rapid postoperative recovery. Therefore, the treatment may be particularly applicable to patients who are only marginally suitable candidates for radical prostatectomy because of age or health and who do not wish to undergo external irradiation. Also, the procedure has the distinct advantage of preserving erectile potency in over 90% of patients. In patients with a reasonable 10- to 15-year life expectancy, the procedure seems to provide somewhat compromised disease-free survival compared to alternative methods.

Combined Au 198 and External Beam Therapy

Interstitial implantation of Au 198 followed by 4,500 rad of external irradiation has provided five- and ten-year survival figures not unlike those achieved with other treatment methods. Seventy-one percent of patients with stage B1 tumors survived one to five years without tumor recurrence. In stage B2 patients, 59% of patients were alive from one to five years after surgery without evidence of disease.[29] However, few patients have received long-term follow-up. Rectal examination has been found to be of limited value in predicting local tumor persistence, and needle biopsies have been positive in 39% of patients, including 30% in whom findings on rectal examination were considered negative.[30]

Iridium 192

Iridium 192 is a pure gamma-emitting isotope with a half-life of 75 days and a half value layer in tissue of 6 cm. Needles are inserted into the prostate through the perineum and afterloading performed. Depending upon the number of needles inserted and the length of time they are left indwelling, from 3,000 to 5,000 rad of irradiation are delivered to the prostate. Supplemental external irradiation is given later. Only a limited number of patients with stage B prostatic cancer have undergone this procedure. However, reported local control and early survival figures have been excellent.[31, 32] Palpable regression of prostatic tumor is rapid after iridium implantation, but rectal complications requiring colostomy have been observed in some patients.

SUMMARY

Discovery of stage B prostatic cancer frequently creates a therapeutic dilemma. A significant number of patients do well for extended periods of time without treatment. On the other hand, detection of stage B prostatic cancer, especially stage B2, is far from an insignificant finding. Tumor progression and death from prostatic cancer occur in a significant number of patients if they are followed for sufficiently long periods of time. Appropriately, it has been pointed out that the impact of treatment upon disease-free survival in patients with stage B prostatic cancer is difficult to assess. Often, good results are attributed to the treatment technique, when the natural history of the disease may be the primary factor that accounts for the excellent five-year survival with virtually any treatment technique. On the other hand, increasing deaths from prostatic cancer are observed with time in all series of patients despite the method of treatment. Nearly one third of patients with stage B prostatic cancer can be expected to develop distant metastatic disease or death from prostatic cancer within ten years.

Stage B prostatic cancer often is detected as an incidental finding in elderly patients. Because of the relatively long disease natural history in most patients, definitive treatment should be withheld in patients with a life expectancy of less than ten years. Although no absolute chronological age can be used as a determinant, patients older than 75 years generally should be spared the morbidity of definitive therapy and be followed with observation alone. Hormonal therapy should be employed if there is any evidence of symptomatic disease progression.

In patients who otherwise have a reasonable life expectancy of ten years or more, aggressive therapy is justified. Long-term disease-free survival has been reported after both radical prostatectomy and external irradiation. Early reports suggested that radical prostatectomy was not suitable for patients with stage B2 prostatic cancer because of a high incidence of extracapsular extension or seminal vesicle invasion. Careful preoperative staging including pelvic lymph node dissection has improved the clinical staging of stage B prostatic cancer, and the majority of patients with stage B2 lesions suitably staged are found to have tumor histologically confined to the prostate after radical prostatectomy. The morbidity of the procedure has been decreased in recent years, and most series report a rate of incontinence of less than 5%. Introduction of a technique for preservation of the periurethral parasympathetic nerve plexus has allowed sexual potency to be maintained in somewhat over half of the patients undergoing radical prostatectomy. Because of these factors, radical prostatectomy has been our preferred form of therapy for most patients with stage B prostatic cancer.

On the other hand, long-term disease-free survival has also been reported after external irradiation, and this remains a reasonable treatment alternative. Analysis of the results of various series is difficult, but five- and ten-year survival figures comparable to radical prostatectomy have been reported. In the only randomized prospective study comparing radical prostatectomy to external irradiation, a statistically significant decrease in the time to evidence of disease progression was found in the radical prostatectomy group. The fact that nearly 50% of patients treated with external irradiation for stage B prostatic cancer have positive postirradiation biopsies is concerning but the impact of this finding on overall survival is yet to be determined.

Introducing further confusion regarding the most appropriate form of treatment for stage B prostatic cancer is the fact that excellent short-term survival figures have been reported for various methods of interstitial irradiation. Disease-free survival, even at five years, seems to be somewhat decreased in patients undergoing iodine 125 implantation, but the low morbidity of the procedure increases its attractiveness.

Often, clinicians state that they "let the patient make the choice" when discussing treatment for stage B prostatic cancer. Such an approach is impractical and probably unfair to patients. Clearly, patients should be well informed of the various treatment options available, and the wishes of the patient are paramount. However, a patient should not be presented with a series of options and asked to decide upon treatment. The clinician's role is to interpret the data, present it in a meaningful manner to patients, be guided in discussions by patient preferences, and make recommendations. In this manner, the most appropriate form of therapy can be selected that provides the greatest chance of prolonged disease-free survival with morbidity that is acceptable for an individual patient.

REFERENCES

1. Murphy GP, Natarajan N, Pontes JE, et al: The National Survey of Prostate Cancer in the United States by the American College of Surgeons. *J Urol* 1982; 127:928–934.
2. Jewett HJ, Bridge RW, Gray GF Jr, et al: The palpable nodule of prostatic cancer. *JAMA* 1968; 203:115–118.
3. Byar DP, Mostofi FK, and VACURG: Carcinoma of the prostate: Prognostic evaluation of certain pathologic features in 208 radical prostatectomies. *Cancer* 1973; 32:5–13.
4. Hanash KA, Utz DC, Cook EN, et al: Carcinoma of the prostate: A fifteen-year follow-up. *J Urol* 1972; 107:450–453.
5. Byar DP, Carle DK: VACURG randomized trial of radical prostatectomy for stages I and II prostate cancer. *Urology* 1981; 17(suppl):7–11.

6. Whitmore WF Jr: Natural history and staging of prostate cancer. *Urol Clin North Am* 1984; 11:205–220.
7. Smith JA Jr, Seaman JP, Gleidman JB, et al: Pelvic lymph node metastasis from prostatic cancer: Influence of tumor grade and stage in 452 consecutive patients. *J Urol* 1983; 130:290–292.
8. Young HH: The early diagnosis and radical cure of carcinoma of the prostate: Being a study of 40 cases and presentation of a radical operation which was carried out in four cases. *Bull Johns Hopkins Hosp* 1905; 16:315–321.
9. Jewett HJ: The present status of radical prostatectomy for stages A and B prostatic cancer. *Urol Clin North Am* 1975; 2:105.
10. Walsh PC, Jewett HJ: Radical surgery for prostatic cancer. *Cancer* 1980; 45:1906–1911.
11. Hodges CV, Pearse HD, Stille L: Radical prostatectomy for carcinoma: 30-year experience in 15-year survivals. *J Urol* 1979; 122:180–182.
12. Gibbons RP, Correa RJ Jr, Brannen GE, et al: Total prostatectomy for localized prostatic cancer. *J Urol* 1984; 131:73.
13. Middleton RG, Smith JA Jr, Melzer RB, et al: Patient survival and local recurrence rate following radical prostatectomy for prostatic cancer. *J Urol* 1986; 136:422–424.
14. Paulson DS, Lin GH, Hinshaw W, and the Uro-Oncology Group: Radical surgery versus radiotherapy for stage A2 and stage B adenocarcinoma of the prostate. *J Urol* 1982; 128:502.
15. Elder JS, Jewett HJ, Wallace PC: Radical perineal prostatectomy for clinical stage B2 carcinoma of the prostate. *J Urol* 1982; 127:704–706.
16. Middleton RG, Smith JA Jr: Radical prostatectomy for stage B2 prostatic cancer. *J Urol* 1982; 127:702–703.
17. Catalona WJ, Fleishmann J, Menon M: Pelvic lymph node status as predictor of extracapsular tumor extension in clinical stage B prostatic cancer. *J Urol* 1983; 129:327–329.
18. Lange PH, Narayan P: Understaging and undergrading of prostate cancer: Argument for postoperative radiation as adjuvant therapy. *Urology* 1983; 21:113.
19. Gibbons RP: Adjuvant radiotherapy following radical prostatectomy: Results and complications. *J Urol* 1986; 135:65.
20. Ray GR, Bagshaw MA, Feiha F: External beam radiation salvage for residual or recurrent local tumor following radical prostatectomy. *J Urol* 1984; 132:926.
21. Jacobson GM, Smith JA Jr, Stewart JR: Postoperative radiation therapy for pathologic stage C prostate cancer, manuscript in preparation.
22. Bagshaw MA, Ray GR, Pistenma DA, et al: External beam radiation therapy of primary carcinoma of the prostate. *Cancer* 1975; 36:723–728.
23. Bagshaw MA, Ray GR, Cox RS: Radiotherapy of prostatic carcinoma: Long- or short-term efficacy. *Urology* 1985; 25:17–23.
24. Pilepich MV, Perez CA, Bauer W: Prognostic parameters in radiotherapeutic management of localized carcinoma of the prostate. *J Urol* 1980; 124:485–487.
25. McGowan DG: Radiation therapy in the management of localized carcinoma of the prostate: A preliminary report. *Cancer* 1977; 39:98–102.
26. Cox JD, Kline RW: The lack of prognostic significance of biopsies after radiotherapy for prostatic cancer. *Semin Urol* 1983; 1:237–242.
27. Scardino PT: The prognostic significance of biopsies after radiotherapy for prostatic cancer. *Semin Urol* 1983; 1:243–251.
28. Schellhammer PF, Ladago LE, El-Mahdi A: Histologic characteristics of prostatic biopsies after iodine 125 implantation. *J Urol* 1980; 23:700–705.

29. Scardino PT, Guerriero WG, Carlton CE Jr: Surgical staging and combined therapy with radioactive gold grain implantation and external irradiation, in Johnson DE, Boileau MN (eds): *Genitourinary Tumor: Fundamental Principles and Surgical Technique.* New York, Grune & Stratton, 1982, pp 75–90.

30. Wheeler TM, Scardino PT: Detailed pathologic review of prostate biopsy following irradiation for carcinoma of the prostate. American Urologic Association Meeting Abstract No. 298, Las Vegas, 1983.

31. Tansey OA, Shanberg AM, Syed AM, et al: Treatment of prostatic carcinoma by pelvic lymphadenectomy, temporary iridium implant and external irradiation. *Urology* 1983; 21:594–598.

32. Miller LS: Afterloading transperineal iridium 192 wire implantation of the prostate. *Radiology* 1979; 13:527–528.

6

Stage C Carcinoma

Stage C prostatic cancer describes locally advanced tumors in which there is no evidence of pelvic lymph node metastasis or extrapelvic disease. Included in this category are tumors that extend beyond the capsule of the prostate to involve the pelvic side wall, seminal vesicle, or bladder base (Fig 6–1). In earlier series, stage C tumors accounted for nearly 40% of the total number of patients seen with prostatic cancer. More recently, the American College of Surgeons survey found stage C tumors at the initial presentation of disease in 15% of patients.[1]

Assignment of a patient to the stage C category usually is based upon digital palpation wherein induration or nodularity is detected extending laterally or superiorly beyond the prostatic capsule. In some patients, distal extension to the membranous urethra is also evident. Prostatic ultrasonography or magnetic resonance imaging (MRI) may detect nonpalpable extracapsular extension in some patients, but the accuracy of these methods of staging has not been fully determined (Fig 6–2). Pathologic stage C prostatic cancer is found in some patients after radical prostatectomy for presumed intracapsular disease when histologic examination of the surgical specimen shows tumor extension beyond the prostatic capsule or invasion into the seminal vesicle.

NATURAL HISTORY OF STAGE C DISEASE

Unlike many stage B tumors, which may remain indolent for long periods of time, stage C prostatic cancer generally is progressive. Only 15% of patients have well-differentiated tumors, and more than 20% have poorly differentiated lesions.[2] Without effective therapy, the five-year survival of patients with stage C tumors is 58%,[3] and 70% show evidence of disease progression. The overall survival of patients at ten years is only 20%.

Seminal vesicle invasion, even if microscopic, implies a poor long-term prognosis.[4] After radical prostatectomy, patients with histologic tumor extension to the seminal vesicles have a poorer prognosis than patients categorized as having stage C disease because of tumor penetration through the prostatic

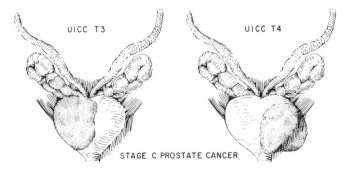

FIG 6–1.
Stage C adenocarcinoma of the prostate includes tumors in which there is extracapsular extension but no distant disease. Tumors often extend superiorly into the base of the seminal vesicle *(left)* or laterally beyond the prostatic capsule *(right)*.

capsule.[5] These factors are of less significance when there is palpable extracapsular tumor extension and this observation may simply reflect differences in tumor bulk.

Approximately one half of patients who are judged to have palpable extracapsular tumor extension are found to have pelvic nodal metastasis after pelvic node dissection and, accordingly, are reclassified as stage D1.[2] Radioimmu-

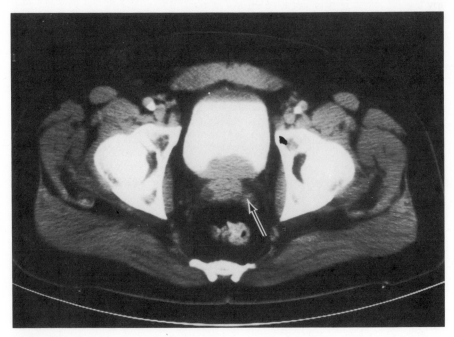

FIG 6–2.
CT scan showing tumor extension to bladder base and left seminal vesicle.

noassay results for serum acid phosphatase may be elevated in some patients with stage C prostatic cancer, although enzymatic acid phosphatase determinations usually are normal. Prostate-specific antigen levels may be elevated in more than half of patients with stage C prostatic cancer.

TREATMENT OPTIONS

Prostatic tumors do not necessarily follow a stage-by-stage progression. Therefore, stage A prostatic cancer may not pass through a detectable phase wherein an intracapsular nodule is palpable before stage C disease is evident. Similarly, small B1 lesions do not necessarily show further intracapsular growth before extracapsular tumor is palpable. Often, progression of stage A or stage B tumors is first detected when palpable induration beyond the prostatic capsule is obvious or metastatic disease is evident. Because of this, even careful follow-up of patients with apparent intracapsular tumors does not necessarily allow detection and intervention prior to the development of stage C disease.

Given the fact that most stage C prostatic cancers are progressive within five years, attempts at definitive therapy are warranted. Although, by definition, tumor has extended beyond the prostatic capsule, the absence of demonstrable tumor beyond the periprostatic region makes effort at definitive local therapy logical. Despite this, curative efforts in most patients with stage C prostatic cancer fail. The event of extracapsular extension generally implies a biologically more virulent tumor than lesions of comparable grade detected at an intracapsular stage. Nevertheless, several treatment options are available.

Surgery

Unlike classic cancer operations, radical prostatectomy produces surgical margins that, even in optimal situations, are precarious. There is no significant amount of soft tissue or fat surrounding the prostate that can be removed along with the surgical specimen. Therefore, the dissection plane follows closely along the prostatic capsule and Denonvilliers' fascia. Accordingly, radical prostatectomy logically seems appropriate only for patients with intracapsular tumors.

Nevertheless, radical prostatectomy has been performed for known stage C tumors in several different series. Schroeder and Belt[6] performed radical perineal prostatectomy in 213 patients with histologic extracapsular extension. Five-year survival was 64%, and local recurrences were seen in 13% of patients. Actuarial survival at 15 years was 20%, but tumor-free survival was only 11%. Most patients received adjunctive hormonal therapy and many had clinical stage B tumors in which extracapsular extension was only microscopic.

Radical prostatectomy for stage C prostatic cancer has also been performed at the Mayo Clinic with apparently good results.[7] However, the addition of hormonal therapy in many patients makes data analysis difficult. Spaulding and Whitmore[8] performed cystoprostatectomy for patients with known tumor extension to the seminal vesicles or bladder base. Justification for this approach was based upon the observation that some patients with bulky local tumor extension die without evidence of distant metastases or have late development of metastasis.[9] Even in patients with histologically negative lymph nodes, long-term results were poor, and this form of therapy does not seem warranted except in highly selected, young patients.

Further evidence that radical prostatectomy generally is not curative for stage C prostatic cancer comes from evaluation of data by Jewett et al.[10] In their series, radical prostatectomy was performed for presumed stage B disease, but histologic examination showed seminal vesicle invasion in some patients. In this group, the long-term prognosis was poor, with a 15-year survival of only 10%. Radical prostectomy alone has been of little benefit in patients with microscopic seminal vesicle invasion. Thus, it seems likely that equally poor long-term results will be obtained when surgery is performed in patients with obvious extracapsular extension.

Even when radical prostatectomy is accepted as an ineffective way to cure stage C prostatic cancer, the operation sometimes has been performed for palliation or prevention of local symptoms.[11] Since surgical margins are likely to be inadequate in most patients, local recurrence may develop in a significant number of patients if followed for sufficient periods of time. Local symptoms generally are manageable by transurethral surgery or hormonal management. Gee and Cole[12] found recurrent obstruction in only 11% of their patients with stage C prostatic cancer. Therefore, there seems little justification for the performance of radical prostatectomy for prevention of possible local problems in the future.

Interstitial Irradiation

Interstitial implantation of radioisotopes into the prostate allows delivery of high doses of radiation to the prostatic tissue. In addition, the isodose curve encompasses the periprostatic tissues. Therefore, brachytherapy with iodine 125, iridium 192, or gold 198 can potentially deliver effective irradiation to tumors that extend beyond the prostatic capsule.

The results of interstitial irradiation with iodine 125 seeds for stage C prostatic cancer have been disappointing. Initially, it was thought that patients with stage C lesions in whom the tumor margins could be reasonably well defined by digital palpation were good candidates for iodine 125 implantation. Analysis of treatment results in these patients has shown poor local control.[13] Biopsy evidence of local tumor persistence or recurrence has been documented in 60% of patients with stage C tumors.[14] Disease-free survival at ten years in stage C patients treated with iodine 125 implantation is 28%. Thus, it seems that the use of interstitial brachytherapy with iodine 125 is applicable only to patients with very limited amounts of palpable extracapsular tumor extension.

There has been less experience with iridium 192, but initial results appear somewhat favorable. The high energy and short half-life of the isotope may be more effective for bulky tumors. Tansey and colleagues[15] found excellent palpable tumor regression in patients and biopsy evidence of local recurrence in only 10% of patients. Further experience and longer follow-up with iridium implantation for stage C prostatic cancer is necessary.

Au 198 with supplemental external irradiation has also been used to treat stage C prostatic cancer.[16] Tumor-free survival at five years has been reported to be 46% and 40% at ten years.[14] However, biopsy-proven local recurrence has been seen in 39% of patients.[17]

Flocks[18] treated stage C prostatic cancer by radical prostatectomy and injection of 2 ml of Au 198 into the bladder base, the urogenital diaphragm, and the vasal stumps. Ten-year tumor-free survival was 67% in patients with negative pelvic nodes and 28% at 25 years.[18] This series and these results have not been reproduced.

External Irradiation

Using external irradiation, portals can be designed that include the entire prostate and periprostatic region. Thus, extracapsular extension of tumor can be encompassed within the radiation field. In addition, a margin of surrounding apparently normal tissue can be included.

When whole-pelvis irradiation is used as treatment of prostatic cancer, doses of around 4,500 rad usually are delivered to the pelvis with a boost to the prostate. Total prostatic and periprostatic doses should be at least 6,500 rad. However, there seems little rationale for including the whole pelvis in the radiation field. First of all, morbidity is increased. If pelvic node dissection has been performed as a staging procedure prior to external irradiation, lower-extremity and genital edema may develop. In addition, the entire bladder is included in the radiation field, increasing the incidence of acute radiation cystitis and long-term radiation changes within the bladder. Furthermore, radiation portals encompassing the entire pelvis include substantial amounts of small bowel, thereby leading to acute radiation enteritis in most patients. Although symptoms usually subside within several months of treatment, long-term complications of radiation enteritis are seen in some patients.

Beyond the increased morbidity, there is little therapeutic benefit in treating the whole pelvis in patients with stage C prostatic cancer. The rationale for such treatment is that radiation may eliminate microscopic tumor deposits in the pelvic lymph nodes. However, numerous studies have shown the inability of external irradiation to prolong disease-free survival in patients with known pelvic lymph node metastasis.[19, 20] On the other hand, if the pelvic nodes histologically are normal, extension of radiation fields probably only increases the morbidity without improving the therapeutic ratio.

Because of these considerations, lymph node staging is useful in patients with clinical stage C prostatic cancer. Since some of these patients develop bulky or gross evidence of lymphadenopathy, CT scanning with skinny-needle aspiration of any abnormal or suspicious lymph nodes should be performed initially. Overall, approximately 25% of patients with stage C prostatic cancer are found to have nodal disease by CT scan. However, actual nodal metastases occur in nearly half of patients with stage C prostatic cancer. Therefore, if CT scanning and needle aspiration fail to confirm lymph node metastases, we generally have proceeded with a surgical lymphadenectomy. Demonstration of nodal metastasis by either method categorizes a patient as having stage D1 disease and indicates that local or regional therapy is unlikely to be of benefit. On the other hand, if the lymph nodes are histologically normal and there is no evidence of extrapelvic disease, the demonstrated tumor burden lies within a radiation field that encompasses the prostate and periprostatic region.

Radiation portals are designed to encompass the entire prostate and a margin surrounding any palpable extension of the tumor for at least 2 cm. In general, the field size is approximately 10 cm by 10 cm. Since the radiation field does not include the whole pelvis, lower-extremity edema usually is not seen even if a surgical lymph node dissection has been performed. In addition, the overall morbidity of this approach is quite low. A total of 6,500 to 7,000 rad is delivered within the radiation field. Localized areas of proctitis may develop but usually resolve promptly. In addition, since the whole bladder is not included in the radiation field, irritative voiding symptoms are decreased and usually resolve completely within six weeks of treatment.

Although the low morbidity of this approach has been demonstrated satisfactorily, the therapeutic efficacy of external irradiation in stage C prostatic cancer remains in question. Bagshaw[21] categorized patients as having "disease limited to the prostate" or "extracapsular extension." Presumably, the latter category comprised patients with stage C tumors. Actuarial five-year survival was 59% in patients with extracapsular extension but decreased to only 30% at ten years.[21]

Cupps and associates[22] reported a 52% five-year survival free of disease in patients with stage C prostatic cancer treated with external irradiation. Ten-year actuarial survival was 63%.

The Uro-Oncology Research Group randomized patients with stage C tumors to whole-pelvic irradiation or observation alone with hormonal therapy upon disease progression. No difference between groups was demonstrable, and 58% of patients on each treatment arm had no detectable progression of disease at five years.[23]

A concern in evaluating the effects of radiation therapy in prostatic cancer is the high incidence of positive biopsy findings after treatment. The demonstrated poor prognosis of patients with positive biopsy results suggests that actuarial survival rates may be inaccurate. Freiha and Bagshaw[24] found positive biopsy results in 60% of patients with stage C tumors more than two years after treatment. Interestingly, 29% of patients with palpably normal prostates had positive biopsy findings.

Undoubtedly, stage C tumors are progressive lesions in most patients and may not respond favorably to external irradiation. However, when careful staging, including lymph node dissection if necessary, fails to demonstrate disease beyond the periprostatic region, external beam irradiation can deliver definitive treatment to all known areas of tumor and, thereby, offer at least a potential for disease control.

Other Treatment Methods

Traditional thinking is that hormonal therapy produces only temporary remissions in patients with prostatic cancer and does not effect a cure. Therefore, endocrine treatment of stage C prostatic cancer is usually not indicated. Occasionally, patients have recurrent symptoms of bladder outlet obstruction, ureteral obstruction, or bleeding from locally extensive tumors even in the absence of distant metastatic disease. In this setting, hormonal therapy should be employed.

The toxic effects of systemic chemotherapy and the overall low objective response rate of prostatic cancer to chemotherapy combine to limit the role of systemic chemotherapy for stage C prostatic cancer. Intra-arterial injection of chemotherapy through the hypogastric artery theoretically has the advantage of delivering high doses of the drugs to the target tissues while limiting systemic toxicity. The superiority of intra-arterial chemotherapy over systemic administration of drugs in treatment of prostatic cancer is unproven. Scardino and Lehane[25] treated eight patients with locally advanced tumors using intra-arterial cis-platinum. Objective responses were observed in three patients. Overall, though, neither systemic nor intra-arterial chemotherapy is indicated for most patients with stage C prostatic cancer.

Microwave hyperthermia has been used for some patients with locally advanced prostatic tumors. Heating beyond 42°C for longer than 30 minutes has been shown to have toxic effect upon some tumor cells. To date, hyperthermia has been used primarily in patients with hormone refractory tumors that are persistent after radiation therapy. Further experience with this modality needs to be obtained before it is considered as a potential form of primary treatment.

MICROSCOPIC EXTRACAPSULAR EXTENSION

The previous discussions in this chapter have referred to patients in whom extracapsular disease extension is detected either by digital rectal examination or imaging procedures such as ultrasonography, CT scanning, or MRI. Another group of patients with stage C prostatic cancer comprises those undergoing radical prostatectomy for presumed stage B tumors in whom microscopic extension beyond the prostatic capsule is detected upon histologic examination. Thus, the tumors are pathologic stage C lesions and surgical margins are inadequate. Local recurrence can be anticipated in a certain percentage of these patients although palpable evidence of recurrence may not be evident for many years. The role of adjuvant irradiation in this setting is controversial. Radiation may reduce the rate of local recurrence but has not resulted in improved survival. Complications including urethral stricture and urinary incontinence may be increased. The incidence of microscopic extracapsular extension and appropriate management of this situation are discussed in greater detail in chapter 4.

SUMMARY

Stage C prostatic cancer is a relatively common finding at the time of disease presentation in many patients. Often, lesions show relatively poor tumor differentiation. Although short-term survival is relatively good, disease-free survival at ten years in patients with stage C tumors is only 20%. Over half of patients with clinical stage C prostatic cancers are found to have pelvic lymph node metastasis. Radical surgery generally is unsatisfactory as a means of long-term cure because surgical margins frequently are inadequate.

Because the short-term prognosis is relatively good, definitive therapy can be withheld in patients with a life expectancy of less than ten years. However, in patients whose life expectancy is greater than ten years, treatment is justified. Because of the high incidence of pelvic node metastasis, lymph node assessment should be performed, first by CT scanning and fine-needle aspiration. If no evidence of lymph node metastasis is detected by this method, surgical lymphadenectomy should be performed. If the pelvic lymph nodes are histologically proven to be free of tumor, irradiation is the preferred form of treatment since radiation fields encompassing the areas of extracapsular extension can be designed. For limited extracapsular extension that can be well defined by digital palpation, interstitial irradiation with iodine 125, iridium 192, or Au 198 may be successful. Most often, external irradiation with treatment to the prostate and periprostatic region is used. Treatment morbidity is acceptable with this approach. The high incidence of posttreatment biopsies is a concern, but ten-year survival rates of 47% have been reported in at least some series.

Although the absolute benefit of this approach in patients with stage C cancer has not been demonstrated, morbidity is relatively low. Hormonal therapy should be withheld unless there is evidence of extrapelvic disease or, occasionally, when recurrent symptoms related to the local tumor develop.

REFERENCES

1. Murphy GP, Natarajan N, Pontes JE, et al: The National Survey of Prostate Cancer in the United States by the American College of Surgeons. *J Urol* 1982; 127:928–934.
2. Smith JA Jr, Seaman JP, Gleidman JB, et al: Pelvic lymph node metastasis from prostatic cancer: Influence of tumor grade and stage in 452 consecutive patients. *J Urol* 1983; 130:290–292.

3. Veterans Administration Cooperative Urological Research Group: Treatment and survival of patients with advanced prostatic cancer. *Surg Gynecol Obstet* 1967; 124:1011–1014.

4. Jewett HJ: The present status of radical prostatectomy for stages A and B prostatic cancer. *Urol Clin North Am* 1975; 2:105.

5. Middleton RG, Smith JA Jr, Melzer RB, et al: Patient survival and local recurrence rate following radical prostatectomy for prostatic cancer. *J Urol* 1986; 136:422–424.

6. Schroeder FH, Belt E: Carcinoma of the prostate: A study of 213 patients with stage C tumors treated by total perineal prostatectomy. *J Urol* 1975; 114:257–260.

7. Zincke H, Fleming TR, Furlow WL, et al: Radical retropubic prostatectomy and pelvic lymphadenectomy for high stage cancer of the prostate. *Cancer* 1978; 47:1901–1910.

8. Spaulding JT, Whitmore WF Jr: Extended total excision of prostatic adenocarcinoma. *J Urol* 1978; 120:188–190.

9. Arnheim FK: Carcinoma of the prostate: A study of the postmortem findings in 176 cases. *J Urol* 1948; 60:599–603.

10. Jewett HJ, Bridge RW, Gray GF Jr, et al: The palpable nodule of prostatic cancer. *JAMA* 1968; 203:115–118.

11. Tomlinson RL, Currie DP, Boyce WH: Radical prostatectomy: Palliation for stage C carcinoma of the prostate. *J Urol* 1977; 117:85–87.

12. Gee WF, Cole JR: Symptomatic stage C carcinoma of prostate: Traditional therapy. *Urology* 1980; 15:335–337.

13. Grossman HB, Batata M, Hilaris B, et al: I-125 implantation of the prostate: Further follow-up of the first 100 cases. *Urology* 1982; 20:591–598.

14. Schellhammer PF, Ladaza LE, El-Mahdi A: Histological characterictics of prostatic biopsies after iodine-125 implantation. *J Urol* 1980; 123:700–705.

15. Tansey LA, Shanberg AM, Syed AM, et al: Treatment of prostatic carcinoma by pelvic lymphadenectomy, temporary iridium-192 implant and external irradiation. *Urology* 1983; 21:594–598.

16. Scardino PT, Guerriero WG, Carlton CE Jr: Surgical staging and combined therapy with radioactive gold grain implantation and external irradiation, in Johnson DE, Boileau MA (eds): *Genitourinary Tumors: Fundamental Principles and Surgical Techniques.* New York, Grune & Stratton, 1982, pp 75–90.

17. Wheeler TM, Scardino PT: Detailed pathologic review of prostate biopsy following irradiation for carcinoma of the prostate. Abstracts of the American Urological Association Meeting, Las Vegas, 1983, No. 298.

18. Flocks RH: The treatment of stage C prostatic cancer with special reference to combined surgical and radiation therapy. *J Urol* 1973; 109:461.

19. Smith JA Jr, Haynes TR, Middleton RG: Impact of external irradiation on local recurrence and disease free survival in patients with pelvic lymph node metastasis from adenocarcinoma of the prostate. *J Urol* 1984; 131:705.

20. Bagshaw MA: Radiotherapy of prostatic cancer: Stanford University Experience, in Kurth KH, Debruyne FM (eds): *Progress and Controversies in Oncologic Urology,* New York, Alan R Liss, 1984, p 493.

21. Bagshaw MA: Radiation therapy of prostatic carcinoma, in Crawford ED, Borden TA (eds): *Genitourinary Cancer Surgery.* Philadelphia, Lee & Febiger, 1982, pp 406–409.

22. Cupps RE, Utz DC, Fleming TR, et al: Definitive radiation therapy for prostatic carcinoma: Mayo Clinic experience. *J Urol* 1980; 124:855–859.

23. Paulson DF, Hodge GB, Hinshaw W: Radiation therapy versus delayed androgen deprivation for stage C carcinoma of the prostate. *J Urol* 1984; 131:901–902.
24. Freiha F, Bagshaw MA: Carcinoma of the prostate: Results of post-irradiation biopsy. *Prostate* 1984; 5:19–72.
25. Scardino PT, Lehane D: Intermittent arterial infusion chemotherapy for advanced, hormonally resistant, radiorecurrent carcinoma of prostate. Abstracts of American Urological Association Annual Meeting, Kansas City, 1982, No. 222.

7

Stage D1 Disease

Although clinicians may be prepared to make recommendations or present treatment options to patients with apparently localized carcinoma of the prostate, the discovery of positive pelvic lymph nodes without evidence of extrapelvic disease frequently creates a confusing situation. Pelvic lymph node metastasis is recognized as a poor prognostic finding, and local or regional therapy does not appear to influence favorably the course of the disease. Nevertheless, expectant therapy alone without therapeutic intervention frequently is poorly accepted by both physicians and patients. The various treatment methods that are sometimes employed for local palliation or potential systemic therapy in patients with stage D1 prostatic cancer are discussed in this chapter, as well as various factors that should influence the selection of therapy.

INCIDENCE OF PELVIC LYMPH NODE METASTASES

In most patients, prostatic cancer seems to follow a pattern of dissemination wherein the pelvic lymph nodes are the first echelon of tumor extension beyond the prostate or periprostatic region. Undoubtedly, distant dissemination to bones or soft tissue occurs in the absence of pelvic lymph node metastasis in some patients, but this appears to be a rare occurrence. Because of this, pelvic lymph node assessment is an important part of staging and selection of therapy for patients with otherwise localized disease (Fig 7–1). Obviously, the status of the pelvic lymph nodes is generally irrelevant in patients with known extrapelvic disease.

The incidence with which pelvic lymph node metastasis occurs related to the clinical stage of the primary tumor is well known. Nodal metastasis is extremely uncommon in stage A1 adenocarcinoma of the prostate gland and probably occurs only in patients in whom clinical evaluation has understaged the tumor.[1] Up to one fourth of patients with stage A2 carcinoma of the prostate are found to have histologic evidence of tumor metastasis within the pelvic lymph nodes. Positive lymph nodes are found in around 12% of patients with small, palpable tumor nodules within the prostate (stage B1) but are detected in some 28% of patients with palpable stage B2 tumors. When there is palpable

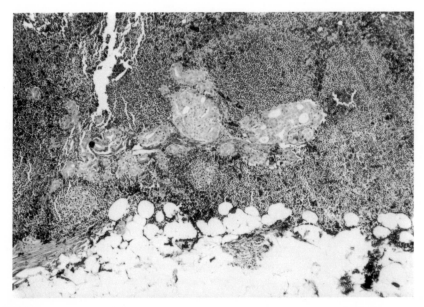

FIG 7–1.
Pelvic lymph node with microscopic metastasis from adenocarcinoma of the prostate. Non-invasive staging techniques such as lymphangiography and computed tomography scanning are unable to detect microscopic nodal disease.

extracapsular extension of tumor to the pelvic side wall or to the seminal vesicles (stage C), approximately one half of patients are found to have pelvic lymph node metastasis.[2]

Tumor grade considered alone also correlates with the incidence of positive pelvic lymph nodes.[3, 4] When patients with clinical stages A2, B, and C are grouped together, only 10% of those with well-differentiated tumors have positive pelvic lymph nodes. Of those with moderately differentiated lesions, about one fourth are found to have pelvic lymph node metastasis, while more than half of those with poorly differentiated tumors have histologic evidence of pelvic node disease.

Even more predictive value is obtained by combining tumor grade and stage. The incidence of pelvic nodal metastatic disease increases with advancing stage, and an even closer correlation is found when grade within stage is considered. Noteworthy are the extremes: only 4% of patients with well-differentiated B1 nodules have positive pelvic lymph nodes compared to over 90% of those with poorly differentiated stage C lesions.

NATURAL HISTORY OF PATIENTS WITH PELVIC LYMPH NODE METASTASIS

The discovery of pelvic lymph node metastasis clearly has adverse prognostic implications. The median time to disease progression is about two years.[5] Disease-free survival at five years is only around 15%.[6,7] Some 75% of patients develop bone metastases within five years, and nearly 40% die of prostatic cancer. The prognosis is only minimally affected by the stage of the primary tumor as the presence of positive pelvic nodes becomes the overriding prognostic factor.

A pertinent issue is the minimal amount of nodal involvement that potentially may be curable by surgery or other methods of local and regional therapy such as external irradiation. It is generally agreed that most patients with gross nodal metastasis have distant although, perhaps, subclinical metastatic disease. However, unless distant metastatic spread occurs simultaneously with pelvic lymph node involvement, there theoretically is a minimum volume of metastatic disease to the pelvic lymph nodes that is curable. In an early analysis of treatment results at Memorial Hospital, it was reported that a volume of nodal disease less than three cubic centimeters inferred no worse prognosis than negative pelvic lymph nodes.[8] Such a finding was at variance with previous studies and the putative pattern of metastatic spread of prostatic cancer. Subsequent analysis at the same institution refuted the initial findings, and the presence of any positive pelvic lymph nodes was found to be a poor prognostic indicator.[9]

Mayo Clinic data have shown a difference in survival between patients with minimal nodal disease compared to those with more extensive amounts. Survival at five years was 91% in patients with two or fewer positive nodes and 60% if five or more nodes were involved.[10] The influence of surgery, hormonal therapy, or both on these results is difficult to determine. Also, it seems probable that longer follow-up will demonstrate that the difference is only in time to disease progression, not in overall survival.

Patients at the University of Utah with positive pelvic lymph nodes have been grouped according to volume of nodal disease[11] (Table 7–1). A variable interval to disease progression was noticeable, with a more favorable short-term prognosis in patients with minimal metastatic disease. At five years, 44% of patients with only a single positive microscopic lymph node were alive without disease progression. Patients with more than one positive microscopic lymph node had only a 27% probability of living five years without development of distant metastatic disease. If gross nodal metastasis was evident, five-year survival without disease progression was only 15% (Table 7–2). While these results reflect variability among the groups, it is likely that these differences are simply related to tumor burden and that virtually all patients are likely to develop evidence of distant metastasis if followed longer. This is further supported by ten-year follow-up among patients that shows a similar overall incidence of recurrence among all groups. These findings are substantiated by numerous other studies that clearly demonstrate a poor long-term prognosis for patients with any evidence of metastatic disease to pelvic lymph nodes, even if it is microscopic and involving only a single lymph node.[2,9,12] Therefore, local or regional therapy alone is unlikely to be of favorable influence in patients with any evidence of nodal metastaic disease.

TABLE 7–1.

Nodal Extent According to Stage of Primary Tumor

| | NODAL EXTENT | | | | | |
| | GROSS, | | MICROSCOPIC, | | SINGLE, | | |
STAGE	NO.	(%)	NO.	%	NO.	(%)	TOTAL
A2	7	(50)	5	(36)	2	(14)	14
B1	4	(27)	6	(40)	5	(33)	15
B2	13	(46)	6	(22)	9	(32)	28
C	9	(56)	5	(31)	2	(13)	16
Total	**33**		**22**		**18**		**73**

TABLE 7–2.

Status at Five Years by Extent of Nodal Disease

	GROSS	MICROSCOPIC	SINGLE
Total no. of patients	33	22	18
Alive, no progression, %	15	27	44
Alive, progressive disease, %	24	27	17
Dead of disease, %	52	37	28
Dead, other causes	9	9	11

TREATMENT OPTIONS FOR STAGE D1 PROSTATIC CANCER

If one accepts the premise that pelvic lymph node metastasis implies distant metastatic disease, then local or regional therapy is destined to fail. On the other hand, there are no currently defined systemic treatments for prostatic cancer that apparently have curative potential. Despite this, a number of treatment modalities have been used, and some favorable, albeit short-term, survival rates have been reported.

Surgical Extirpation

Radical surgery for stage D1 prostatic cancer has provided mixed results. Spaulding and Whitmore[13] reported pelvic node dissection and cystoprostatectomy in 18 patients with nodal metastasis from prostatic cancer. Only two patients (11%) lived five years free of tumor; one of these died of cancer at 13 years. Flocks[14] combined pelvic lymphadenectomy, radical prostatectomy, and Au 198 instillation of the bladder neck. Although 88% of patients lived five years, only 12% survived ten years after surgery. Paulson[12] found progression within 42 months in all of 11 patients with positive nodes undergoing lymphadenectomy and radical prostatectomy. Zincke and Utz[10] reported a five-year nonprogression rate of only 18% in 52 node-positive patients treated with radical prostatectomy and pelvic lymphadenectomy but no early hormonal therapy.

These data appear to demonstrate no favorable influence of radical surgery alone on time to progression or overall survival of prostate cancer patients with positive nodes. Sometimes, radical surgery is performed on the premise that symptoms of local recurrence are prevented by surgery. However, local symptoms usually are manageable by more conservative methods. Nearly half of patients receiving no treatment to the primary tumor live five years without significant local symptoms.[6]

External Irradiation

A common treatment for patients with stage D1 prostatic cancer is external irradiation. Historically, extended field size has been used with portals encompassing the whole pelvis as well as the para-aortic lymph nodes. Evidence has shown that treatment of para-aortic lymph nodes is not fruitful, but pelvic irradiation continues to be used in some patients with identified nodal metastases.

For the same reasons that the curative potential of radical prostatectomy is limited in patients with histologically proven pelvic lymph node metastases, external irradiation is likely to fail. Although extended radiation fields can be used, it remains a method of regional therapy for a disease that is likely systemic. Nevertheless, the concept that external irradiation is capable of "sterilizing" lymph node metastasis has led to its use in stage D1 prostatic cancer.

Most often, approximately 4,500 rad is delivered to the pelvis with a prostatic boost to between 6,500 and 7,000 rad. Radiation cystitis and enteritis usually are transient, but prolonged severe symptoms are seen in up to 10% of patients. Also of significance is the fact that lower-extremity edema occurs commonly if a complete surgical lymph node dissection has been performed. Although the incidence of edema after irradiation is somewhat less with modified pelvic node dissection, edema remains a problem when pelvic radiation and surgical lymphadenectomy are combined. Edema is a lesser problem in patients in whom pelvic lymph node metastasis is confirmed by lymphangiography or CT scanning with skinny-needle biopsy.

Results of external irradiation for patients with stage D1 prostatic cancer generally show no apparent benefit in overall survival or disease-free interval.[15] Bagshaw et al.[16] found tumor recurrence in 50 (82%) of 61 patients with histologically proven pelvic node metastasis treated with external irradiation. The median follow-up was seven years. The Uro-Oncology Research Group randomized patients with positive nodes to therapy with external beam irradiation or delayed endocrine treatment.[17] Although there was a mild increase in the time to progression in irradiated patients, overall survival at five years was equal between groups.

We analyzed retrospectively patients with positive nodes treated with ex-

ternal irradiation or observation alone. Both groups received delayed endocrine therapy if there was evidence of disease progression. At five years, 48%
of patients treated with irradiation were alive compared with 53% of patients
in the observation group. Distant disease had developed within five years in
76% of irradiated patients and in 65% of the observation group.[6] These differences are not significant and are further evidence that external irradiation imparts no apparent survival benefit in patients with positive nodes (Table 7–3).

Another potential reason for using external irradiation in patients with
proven pelvic lymph node metastasis is the possibility that treatment may prevent local symptoms. Since most patients with metastatic prostatic cancer have
tumors that have demonstrated a higher malignant potential based simply on
the fact that nodal dissemination has occurred, it is not surprising to discover
that local control rates in this group are lower than those achieved with external irradiation for intracapsular tumors. In Bagshaw's series, results of post-
treatment biopsies of the prostate were positive in 69% of patients.[18]

We compared local symptoms in patients with stage D1 prostatic cancer
treated by external irradiation or observation alone. Over half of the patients
who had not received irradiation or any other form of treatment to the local
prostatic tumor developed symptoms related to local tumor progression within
five years. Bladder outlet obstructive symptoms, ureteral obstruction, perineal
pain, or recurrent bleeding were seen in 65% of these patients, but the others
had no symptoms related to the local tumor despite the absence of treatment.
Slightly less than half the irradiated patients remained symptom free while
51% developed local symptoms because of tumor persistence and local progression (Table 7–4).

Based on these data, there is little therapeutic basis for a recommendation
of external irradiation in patients with pelvic lymph node metastasis from pros-

TABLE 7–3.

Survival at Five Years by Stage of Primary Lesion in Patients With
Positive Nodes

	STAGE				TOTAL NO. OF PATIENTS (%)
	A1	B1	B2	C	
Pelvic irradiation					
Alive, free of disease	1	4	2	1	8 (17)
Alive, with disease	3	4	5	3	15 (32)
Dead of disease	3	3	7	6	19 (40)
Dead, other causes	2	0	3	0	5 (11)
Total	**9**	**11**	**17**	**10**	**47 (100)**
No irradiation					
Alive, free of disease	0	1	3	1	5 (29)
Alive, with disease	2	1	0	1	4 (24)
Dead of disease	1	0	3	2	6 (35)
Dead, other causes	0	1	1	0	2 (12)
Total	**3**	**3**	**7**	**4**	**17 (100)**

TABLE 7–4.

Local Symptoms Within Five Years*

	PELVIC IRRADIATION	NO IRRADIATION
Bladder outlet obstruction	11	6
Ureteral obstruction	5	2
Bleeding	4	1
Perineal pain	4	2
Total, No. (%)	**24** (51)	**11** (65)

*Table showing local symptoms within five years in patients with stage D1 prostatic cancer treated with pelvic irradiation compared to patients receiving no primary therapy to the prostate. No substantial difference between the two groups is observed.

tatic cancer. Numerous studies show no difference in long-term survival. Palliative therapy by irradiation is not necessary in half the patients and is unsuccessful in most of the remaining ones.

Hormonal Therapy

Traditional thinking is that hormonal therapy provides palliation and, perhaps, a longer interval to disease progression in patients with prostatic cancer but is not curative. Additionally, some evidence has suggested that delayed institution of treatment is as effective as early hormonal therapy. Application of these concepts to stage D1 prostatic cancer leads to the treatment philosophy that hormonal therapy should be withheld until patients develop extrapelvic disease or recurrent local symptoms. Presumably, a patient with stage D1 prostatic cancer who begins hormonal therapy immediately would have a longer interval to disease progression than a patient simply observed and not treated with endocrine therapy. Once disease progression occurs, institution of hormonal therapy in the latter patient would likely produce a temporary clinical remission, while the patient already receiving hormonal therapy would have no response to subsequent endocrine manipulation. Overall symptom free survival would be equal between both patients.

These traditional concepts have been challenged, and there is some enthusiasm for early institution of hormonal therapy in patients. There is some experimental evidence suggesting a salutary role for early hormonal treatment based upon the concept that less tumor heterogeneity and, therefore, fewer hormonally resistant cells are present in earlier stages of the disease.[19] Much of the clinical data supporting this approach comes from the Mayo Clinic.[10] Although the patient series is large, it is nonhomogeneous, with variable follow-up. Nevertheless, orchiectomy at the time of radical prostatectomy in patients with proven lymph node metastases has provided actuarial survival rates of 85% and 68% at five and ten years, respectively. Patients treated by radical prostatectomy with delayed orchiectomy had a nonprogression rate of only 18% at five years. Thus, the contribution of orchiectomy to these data seems clear. Interestingly, in a smaller subset of patients treated with early DES instead of orchiectomy, nonprogression rates were similar to nonhormonally treated patients.

These results at least raise the possibility that early hormonal therapy may be of benefit in node-positive patients. However, the variable and relatively short follow-up in these patients should be emphasized. Reported survival figures are actuarial, and only one third of the patients had been at risk for five years or more. Longer follow-up may demonstrate that immediate orchiectomy simply prolongs the interval to disease progression without influencing overall survival.

Chemotherapy

Although the results of cytotoxic chemotherapy for prostatic cancer generally have been disappointing, most trials have been conducted in patients with hormone refractory metastatic disease and a large tumor burden. It has been suggested that earlier institution of chemotherapy, perhaps in an adjuvant fashion, may improve results. On the other hand, the rarity with which complete responses are observed after chemotherapy in stage D2 suggests that the currently available cytotoxic agents have little potential for cure when used in an adjuvant fashion. Arguments in favor of adjuvant chemotherapy are based primarily on the belief that treatment may be more effective with less tumor bulk and that patients with early-stage disease will tolerate cytotoxic chemotherapy better.

Only extremely limited data about the use of cytotoxic chemotherapy for stage D1 prostatic cancer have been accumulated. DeVere White and colleagues[20] used adjuvant chemotherapy consisting of cyclophosphamide (Cytoxan) (750 mg/sq m) and doxorubicin (Adriamycin) (50 mg/sq m) to a total of 450 mg/sq m) in 12 patients with stage D1 disease. All patients had undergone either interstitial implantation of I 125 in the prostate or radical prostatectomy. With a short period of follow-up (12 to 36 months) four had disease progression an average of 15 months after treatment. The small numbers and short follow-up allow no conclusions to be drawn, but toxic reactions were minimal. The National Prostatic Cancer Project randomized patients treated with external irradiation to no additional therapy or adjuvant Cytoxan.[21] Although the chemotherapy was relatively well tolerated, no difference in time to disease progression or overall survival was seen.

Further studies of early chemotherapy in patients with stage D1 prostate cancer are indicated. However, the limited data available and the general lack of objective response seen in patients with more widespread disease suggest that a substantial improvement in survival is unlikely with currently available agents. At this time, there seems little justification for the use of adjuvant chemotherapy on a routine basis in patients with stage D1 prostatic cancer.

TREATMENT OF STAGE D0 DISEASE

Another category of prostatic cancer deserving consideration is the recently described D0 stage. Included in this group are patients without demonstrable metastatic disease to pelvic lymph nodes or distant sites but with an elevated serum acid phosphatase level. Depending on the method of assay, an elevated serum acid phosphatase level generally is indicative of extracapsular tumor, usually in bone or pelvic lymph nodes. In the D0 category, however, the only evidence of extraprostatic tumor is the elevated serum acid phosphatase level. Questions arise, then, regarding whether these patients should be considered to have metastatic disease or whether they should be treated as if their tumor is localized.

Often, patients initially are categorized as having D0 disease based upon a normal bone scan and a CT scan or lymphangiogram showing no evidence of pelvic nodal disease. If these patients are subjected to a surgical pelvic lymphadenectomy, the majority will be found to have microscopic evidence of lymph node metastasis. Strictly defined, stage D0 includes only patients with histologic evidence of normal pelvic lymph nodes. Whitesel and associates[22] demonstrated a poor prognosis for patients with histologically negative pelvic lymph nodes and an elevated serum acid phosphatase level compared with those with normal lymph nodes and acid phosphatase determinations. Similarly, Scardino et al.[23] found that only one of 28 patients with an elevated acid phosphatase level but otherwise localized disease lived 11 years free of disease.

Clearly, an elevated serum acid phosphatase level is a poor prognostic sign even in the face of a normal bone scan and normal pelvic lymph nodes. Considering this, the primary therapeutic question is whether these patients should be considered to have systemic disease or be treated as if the tumor is localized. Although the poorer prognosis of these patients is recognized, we generally have not excluded them from definitive therapy when lymph nodes are histologically normal and the acid phosphatase evaluation is modest. A small subset of patients may have serum acid phosphatase elevation in the absence of extracapsular disease. No large patient series are available to justify this approach but, if patients are otherwise good candidates for treatment, exclusion from therapy on the basis of a serum acid phosphatase elevation alone seems overly restrictive.

SUMMARY

Identification of stage D1 prostatic cancer in an otherwise healthy patient presents a therapeutic dilemma. In the absence of effective therapy, long-term prognosis is poor and 75% of patients develop skeletal metastasis within five years. Although differences in time to disease progression are demonstrable depending on the number or volume of nodal metastases, all patients probably have systemic disease. Therefore, local or regional therapy is destined to fail. Radical surgery alone in this setting seems unjustified. External irradiation delivered to either wide or more limited fields has not favorably influenced survival. More than two thirds of patients treated with external irradiation have had persistence of biopsy-proven tumor in the prostate, and there has been no difference in the frequency or severity of local symptoms between irradiated and nonirradiated patients.

In general, if positive nodes are demonstrated by nonsurgical staging maneuvers such as a CT scan or lymphangiography and are histologically confirmed by needle aspiration, radical surgery is not recommended. Similarly, if grossly positive nodes are encountered at pelvic lymphadenectomy, no role for further surgery has been established. Frozen-section detection of microscopic nodal disease at the time of pelvic lymphadenectomy likely identifies a patient who will not benefit from radical surgery alone. Surgical debulking has been shown to be of minimal or no benefit in most human carcinomas, and there is no evidence of any favorable effects on prostatic cancer.

On the other hand, systemic therapy for prostatic cancer that is capable of improving survival probably does not exist. Cytotoxic chemotherapy has produced minimal objective responses in patients with extrapelvic metastases, and current agents are unlikely to be effective in an adjuvant setting. The putative mechanism of action of hormonal therapy suggests that overall survival will be similar whether treatment is initiated early or late. In direct and striking contrast to this concept are the data from the Mayo Clinic demonstrating improved disease-free survival by the combination of radical prostatectomy and immediate orchiectomy in patients with histologically proven stage D1 disease.

For most patients, the most logical clinical approach to stage D1 disease is to spare the patient the morbidity of treatment that is unlikely to be of benefit. The morbidity and expense of radical prostatectomy or external irradiation and their inherent inability in influence favorably systemic disease mitigate against their use on a routine basis. Although endocrine therapy without significant side effects other than decreased libido and impotence is available, early hormonal therapy alone has not been shown to be of benefit. Further studies of the effects of early endocrine treatment are needed. In the absence of treatment that has been shown definitively to improve survival, most patients are probably best treated by judicious observation alone, with institution of hormonal therapy when disease progression is evident.

REFERENCES

1. Parfitt HE, Smith JA Jr, Middleton RG: Accuracy of staging in A1 carcinoma of the prostate. *J Urol* 1983; 129:763.
2. Donohue RE, Fauver HE, Whitesel JG, et al: Prostatic carcinoma: Influence of tumor grade on results of pelvic lymphadenectomy. *Urology* 1981; 17:435–440.
3. Smith JA Jr, Seamon JP, Gleidman JB, et al: Pelvic lymph node metastases from prostatic cancer: Influence of tumor grade and stage. *J Urol* 1983; 130:290–292.

4. Paulson DF, Piserchia PV, Gardner W: Predictors of lymphatic spread in prostatic adenocarcinoma: Uro-Oncology Research Group Study. *J Urol* 1980; 123:697–699.
5. Kramer SA, Spahr J, Brendler CB, et al: Experience with Gleason's histopathologic grading in prostatic cancer. *J Urol* 1980; 124:223–225.
6. Smith JA Jr, Middleton RG: Impact of external irradiation on disease-free survival and local symptoms in patients with pelvic lymph node metastases from prostatic cancer. *J Urol* 1984; 131:705–708.
7. DeVere White R: Radiation and chemotherapy for stage D1 prostatic cancer. *Semin Urol* 1983; 1:261–267.
8. Barzell W, Bean MA, Hilaris BS, et al: Prostatic adenocarcinoma: Relationship of grade and local extent to the pattern of metastases. *J Urol* 1977; 118:278–282.
9. Grossman HB, Batata M, Hilaris B, et al: I-125 implantation for carcinoma of the prostate: Further follow-up of the first 100 cases. *Urology* 1982; 20:591–598.
10. Zincke H, Utz DC: Radical surgery for stage D1 prostate cancer. *Semin Urol* 1983; 4:253–260.
11. Smith JA Jr, Middleton RG: Implications of volume of nodal metastases in patients with adenocarcinoma of the prostate. *J Urol* 1985; 133:617–619.
12. Paulson DF: The prognostic role of lymphadenectomy in adenocarcinoma of the prostate. *Urol Clin North Am* 1980; 7:615–622.
13. Spaulding JT, Whitmore WF Jr: Extended total excision of prostatic adenocarcinoma. *J Urol* 1980; 120:188–190.
14. Flocks RH: The treatment of stage C prostatic cancer with special reference to combined surgical and radiation therapy. *J Urol* 1973; 109:461–463.
15. Batata MA, Hilaris BS, Chu FCH, et al: Radiation therapy in adenocarcinoma of the prostate with pelvic lymph node involvement on lymphadenectomy. *Int J Radiol Oncol Biol Phys* 1980; 6:149–153.
16. Bagshaw MA, Ray GB, Cox RS: Radiotherapy of prostatic carcinoma: Long- or short-term efficacy. *Urology* 1985; 25 (suppl):17–23.
17. Paulson DF, Cline WA Jr, Koefoot RB Jr: Extended field radiation therapy versus delayed hormonal therapy in node positive prostatic adenocarcinoma. *J Urol* 1982; 127:935–939.
18. Stamey TA: Cancer of the prostate. *Monographs in Urology* 1982; 3:67–93.
19. Coffey DS, Benson MC: Prostate cancer research: Current concepts and controversies. *Semin Urol* 1983; 1:323–330.
20. De Vere White R, Babaian RK, Krikorian J: Adjuvant chemotherapy for stage D1 adenocarcinoma of prostate. *Urology* 1983; 21:270–272.
21. Gibbons RP, for the National Prostatic Cancer Project: Cooperative trials of single and combined agent protocols. *Urology* 1981; 17(suppl):48–52.
22. Whitesel JA, Donohue RE, Mani JN, et al: Acid phosphatase—its influence in pelvic lymph node dissection. Abstracts of the American Urologic Association Meeting, Kansas City, 1982, abstract No. 236.
23. Scardino PT, Seale C, Carlton CE Jr: The prognostic significance of enzymatic prostatic acid phosphatase in clinically localized prostatic cancer. *J Urol* 1984; 131:158A.

8

Endocrine Treatment

The partial androgen dependence of most prostatic cancers has been recognized since the pioneering work of Huggins and Hodges in 1941.[1] It was reasoned that, since normal prostatic cancer cells were partially androgen dependent, prostatic carcinoma should retain some of the requirement for androgenic stimulation. The demonstrated response in most patients to orchiectomy or estrogen administration, as well as the reversal of these changes with exogenous testosterone administration, verified these thoughts. Numerous studies since then have confirmed their results. Over 45 years later, endocrine manipulation with suppression of either androgen production or blockade of cellular androgenic effects remains the most effective and commonly employed treatment for metastatic carcinoma of the prostate (Fig 8–1).

PHYSIOLOGY

The aim of hormonal manipulation in the treatment of patients with prostatic cancer is to deprive the tumor cells of androgens or their byproducts. Any treatment that decreases production or interferes with delivery of androgens to the cell is likely to produce an objective and subjective response in most patients with prostatic cancer. The physiologic delivery of androgens to tumor cells is incompletely understood, but there are multiple points along the pathway between production and metabolism at which the cycle may be broken.

The major circulating androgen in men is testosterone, 90% of which is produced by the testes. Testosterone released from the testes is regulated by the hypothalamic-pituitary-gonadal axis. Stimulated by the neurotransmitter norepinephrine, gonadotropin-releasing hormone is released in a pulsatile fashion from the median eminence of the hypothalamus. In turn, luteinizing hormone (LH) and follicle-stimulating hormone (FSH) are produced by the anterior pituitary. Direct action of LH upon the Leydig cells of the testis causes the release of testosterone into the bloodstream. Most circulating testosterone is bound to blood proteins, either albumin or testosterone estrogen binding

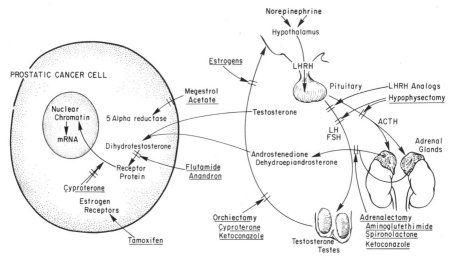

FIG 8–1.
Diagram showing hypothalamic-pituitary-gonadal axis as well as the intracellular metabolism of androgens. Multiple points of entry into the pathway between androgen production and metabolism are available.

globulin, a specific sex steroid binding protein. The functionally active form of testosterone is the approximately 3% that remains unbound to protein.[2]

Portions of the intracellular metabolism of male sex steroids are well understood; others are not. Unbound testosterone diffuses passively into the cytoplasm of the cell and is converted into dihydrotestosterone (DHT) by the enzyme 5-alpha-reductase. DHT in the cytoplasm is bound to a receptor protein and then to the DNA of nuclear chromatin. Messenger RNA is produced and codes several proteins for metabolic function essential for a prostatic acinar cell.

Although most circulating androgen in men is of testicular origin, a relatively small amount of androgen is produced by the adrenal gland. The steroids androstenedione and dehydroepiandrosterone are released by the adrenal gland in response to ACTH from the anterior pituitary gland. Both are relatively weak androgens compared to testosterone or dihydrotestosterone and are almost completely bound by serum protein. Androstenedione and dehydroepiandrosterone are partially converted to testosterone and DHT in androgen-responsive tissue such as skin and hair follicles. The ability of adrenal androgens to promote secondary sexual characteristics through intracellular conversion to DHT is demonstrated in pathologic conditions such as Cushing's syndrome, idiopathic hirsutism, adrenal hyperplasia, or adrenal tumors. In normal physiologic situations, the role of adrenal androgen production in the development and maintenance of masculinization seems to be minimal. The contribution of adrenal androgens to the growth of prostatic cancer cells, in either the presence or absence of testicular production of testosterone, is uncertain.

The majority of prostatic cancer cells are at least partially androgen dependent. The putative explanation is that prostatic cancer cells are derived from a heterogeneous population with a variable metabolic requirement for androgen. Thus, tumors composed primarily of cells that are androgen dependent respond most favorably to hormonal manipulation. Tumor relapse in hormonally treated patients may result from the development of hormone resistance in previously sensitive cells or the emergence of androgen-independent cells, although most theories favor the latter hypothesis. At any rate, effective endocrine treatment of prostatic cancer depends upon the ability to block either the production or delivery of androgens to prostatic cancer cells.

EFFECTS OF HORMONAL THERAPY

Some 80% of patients with prostatic cancer can be expected to have a favorable response to adequate hormonal therapy. There is no apparent difference in the incidence or response between any treatment that adequately suppresses testosterone to the castrate range (less than 50 ng/dl) or effectively blocks the intracellular metabolism or uptake of androgens. Recently, there has been renewed interest in the possibility that further reduction in serum androgens by blocking adrenal androgenic effects may improve the response (see section on total androgen suppression). Presumably, the approximately 20% of patients who do not respond to hormonal therapy have androgen-insensitive tumors, although it has been suggested that these patients have tumor cells that are exquisitely androgen sensitive and stimulated by the low levels of circulating androgen that remain after ablation of testicular sources of testosterone.[4]

The typical endocrine response in most patients is both rapid and profound. A decrease in tumor cell mass occurs. In patients with measurable or palpable soft-tissue metastases, this objective response can easily be assessed (Fig 8–2). The objective decrease in tumor size in patients with bone metastases is less easily documented, although bone scans may show considerable improvement several months after initiation of endocrine therapy and occasionally revert to normal (Fig 8–3). Serial digital palpations of the prostate often show that a palpable nodule or area of induration becomes less distinct and smaller. The normal prostatic acinar cells also undergo involution with androgen deprivation. Thus, the prostatic fossa often is palpable as a rather scaphoid, flat area with indistinct induration.

Due to the objective reduction in tumor size, symptomatic response follows. Most patients with bone pain, even those with severe pain requiring narcotics, often receive total or nearly complete relief of their pain. Recalcification of osteolytic metastases may be seen on skeletal roentgenograms.

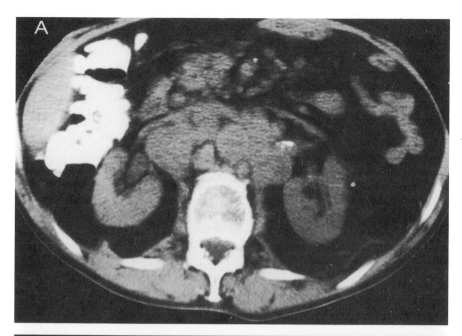

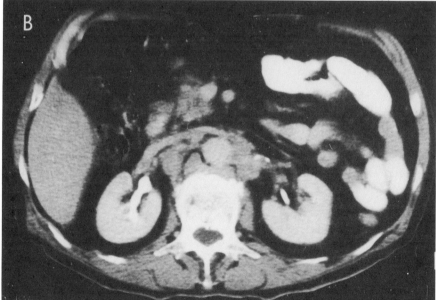

FIG 8–2.
A, retroperitoneal adenopathy at level of renal hilum before treatment. **B,** six weeks after hormonal therapy, marked objective decrease in size of adenopathy is evident. After cytotoxic chemotherapy, objectively measurable responses are unusual.

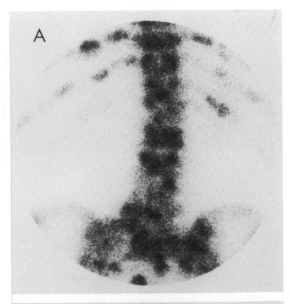

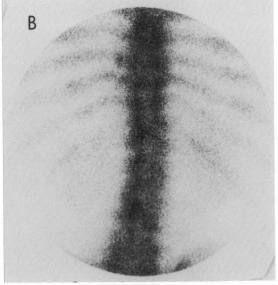

FIG 8–3.
A, bone scan showing diffuse metastatic involvement of pelvis, lumbar spine, and ribs. **B,** three months after institution of hormonal therapy with an LHRH analog, marked improvement is evident with a decrease in the number and intensity of metastatic foci.

Lower-extremity edema caused by venous compression or decreased lymphatic outflow from pelvic nodal metastases may improve if venous thrombosis is not present. In as many as three fourths of patients with unilateral or bilateral ureteral obstruction from subtrigonal tumor extension, hydronephrosis improves. Finally, involution of the prostate produces an improvement in obstructive voiding symptoms and may allow up to half of patients in urinary retention eventually to void spontaneously.

Duration of Response

Hormonal therapy does not cure prostatic cancer, and the favorable effects are only temporary. The duration of response is variable and unpredictable. Most clinicians have anecdotal stories of patients with apparent responses for many years after hormonal manipulation. However, the average duration of remission in patients with metastatic carcinoma of the prostate is around 18 months.

Relapse after a previously satisfactory endocrine response may be heralded by a number of clinical, laboratory, or radiographic findings. Whether relapse indicates lack of hormonal response in cells that were previously androgen sensitive or simply the emergence of androgen-insensitive cells that were present at the initiation of treatment is unclear. At any rate, some sites of metastatic disease may show clear evidence of progression while others remain unchanged and in apparent good remission.

Often, areas of increasing bone pain are the first sign of relapse of prostatic cancer after hormonal therapy. Serum acid phosphatase usually rises above maximally suppressed values. A bone scan may simply show increasing density at areas of known metastatic disease but, often, new lesions are detected. Prostate-specific antigen (PSA) recently has been found to be a highly sensitive marker for progressive disease or relapse.

Timing of Endocrine Therapy

The time point at which endocrine therapy should be instituted in patients with prostatic cancer depends upon an interpretation of what can be accomplished with endocrine therapy as well as a philosophic approach to treatment. Issues of importance are whether duration of response is influenced by tumor bulk. It is only logical that, if the time at which hormonal therapy is employed does not influence patient survival or response duration, endocrine treatment should be withheld until disease symptoms develop. Unfortunately, a definitive answer to these issues is not available. The influence of hormonal therapy on overall patient survival can only be inferred from historical series since withholding endocrine therapy until patient death would no longer be ethical. Thus, the nonrandomized series from the 1950s as well as the studies of the Veterans Administration Cooperative Research Group have had a profound impact on current thinking regarding the timing of endocrine therapy.

In 1946, Vest and Frazier[5] as well as Nesbit and Plumb[6] compared survival of patients treated with estrogens or orchiectomy to control patients from the prehormonal period. Both studies suggested that survival was prolonged in hormonally treated patients although other significant advances occurred during that time period, including the advent of effective antibiotics. Nesbit and Baum[7] conducted a multi-institutional cooperative study and concluded that endocrine therapy prolonged survival for all patients with prostatic cancer and that it should be instituted at the time of first diagnosis.

The most elaborate studies of the effects of hormone treatment in prostatic cancer were conducted by the Veterans Administration Cooperative Urologic Research Group (VACURG). Study I randomized patients with early-stage disease (A or B) to radical prostatectomy plus placebo or radical prostatectomy plus 5 mg of diethylstilbestrol (DES).[8] Patients receiving 5 mg of DES daily had a significant increase in cardiovascular deaths. Patients with stage 3 or 4 (stage C or D) tumors received either placebo or some form of hormonal therapy. Patients randomized to placebo appeared to have an overall survival similar to those receiving endocrine therapy. However, the substantial majority of patients initially randomized to placebo received some form of endocrine therapy at the time of disease progression.[9]

Several conclusions can be drawn from this study. First, high-dose estrogens have an adverse effect on overall patient survival. Also, there appears to be no significant difference in overall patient survival whether endocrine therapy is instituted early in the disease process or whether treatment is delayed until progressive disease is evident.

Despite these data, there has been a tendency for earlier institution of hormonal therapy in recent years. Endocrine treatment has been promoted as adjuvant therapy to radical prostatectomy or early institution of chemotherapy. In both situations, it is implied that hormonal therapy may not simply prolong patient survival but may actually increase cure rates.

Given the conflicting information that exists, various opinions can be obtained regarding the appropriate timing of hormonal therapy in the treatment of patients with prostatic cancer. Nevertheless, several practical conclusions can be drawn and recommendations made. First of all, it is likely that hormonal therapy does prolong survival in some patients. However, this is somewhat of a moot point since all patients with progressive prostatic cancer should receive some form of adequate endocrine therapy at some point in their disease. The time at which endocrine treatment is employed is likely not a critical decision. Early institution of hormonal therapy will prolong the interval until metastatic disease develops but, once metastases are evident, rapid progression can be anticipated. On the other hand, if endocrine treatment is withheld until symptomatic metastatic disease occurs, introduction of hormonal treatment likely will produce an objective and subjective response. Overall patient survival is probably unaffected whether treatment is employed early or late. In addition, patients receiving delayed therapy are spared the potential side effects of hormonal treatment for the months or years during which therapy is withheld.

In general, it has been our recommendation that hormonal therapy be withheld until there is evidence of disease progression. Thus, a patient with an apparently localized tumor with evidence of increasing local tumor size, recurrent bladder outlet obstruction, or ureteral obstruction should receive hormonal therapy. Likewise, a patient who previously had no evidence of distant metastatic disease who develops extrapelvic metastases usually receives endocrine therapy at the time of recognition of metastatic disease even if he is asymptomatic. The interval between detection of metastases and development of symptoms in patients with obviously progressive tumor is slight, and there is little to be gained by withholding treatment at that point. On the other hand, treatment can be safely deferred in patients with metastatic disease until there is evidence of further progression or the development of symptomatic metastases. Further studies on the role of early hormonal therapy are warranted.

METHODS OF HORMONAL THERAPY

There are a number of points of entry into the hypothalamic pituitary gonadal axis and the intracellular metabolism of androgens that allow either a block in androgen synthesis or that interfere with intracellular metabolic processes.

Various surgical procedures are designed to ablate the output of testosterone from the testes or remove adrenal androgen sources. In addition, surgical ablation of the pituitary gland effectively eliminates gonadotropins and adrenal corticostimulating hormone. Various drugs are capable of reproducing these surgical effects. Finally, new classes of compounds act at the cellular level to interfere with the metabolic conversion of serum androgens.

Conventional Hormonal Therapy

Orchiectomy

Surgical orchiectomy removes the primary source of circulating testosterone in men and a rapid fall in measurable serum levels of testosterone results. Within 12 hours, testosterone is suppressed to the castrate range, generally accepted to be less than 50 ng/dl.[10] Since Huggins and Hodges' original work, orchiectomy has endured as the most commonly employed form of hormonal therapy for prostatic cancer patients.

Orchiectomy is a simple and safe surgical procedure. The operation can be accomplished under a local anesthetic, and postoperative pain is minimal. Most often, the entire testis is removed along with the epididymis, but a subcapsular orchiectomy can be performed. The blood clot and fibrosis that fill the tunica albuginea after a subcapsular orchiectomy may mimic a normal testis. In addition, the epididymis may be left in site. An alternative is to place silicone testicular prostheses after orchiectomy. These maneuvers rarely seem necessary, and most patients who accept the procedure do not suffer any significant psychologic problems because of the empty scrotum.

As with all hormonal therapies that suppress serum levels of testosterone, most patients become impotent within a few months of orchiectomy. Associated with the erectile dysfunction is a decreased libido. Some generalized loss of facial and body hair occurs. Vasomotor hot flashes develop in some patients.

These may be suppressed by low doses of estrogen (0.25 mg of DES daily). Some antihypertensives and ergotamine containing compounds have also been reported to be effective in suppressing the hot flashes.

Estrogens

The most frequently used alternative hormonal treatment in patients who refuse orchiectomy has been administration of estrogens. Most often, DES is administered orally. Although there is some evidence of a direct effect of DES on the testis,[11] the accepted mechanism of action of estrogens is feedback inhibition of pituitary secretion of LH. In addition, estrogens may increase circulating levels of sex steroid binding globulin, thereby reducing the amount of unbound testosterone.

The side effects of oral estrogens have been well documented. Painful gynecomastia is frequent. Pretreatment breast irradiation may not prevent the breast enlargement but often is effective in reducing the pain. Pedal edema is common, and nausea and vomiting occur in some patients. Of greater concern is the increased incidence of deep venous thrombosis and cardiovascular deaths associated with both the 3-mg and the 5-mg daily dosing schemes. The risk of thromboembolic complication seems to be lessened with a 1 mg/day dose, but serum levels of testosterone may be incompletely suppressed.[12]

LHRH ANALOGS

As recently as 1971, Schally and co-workers[13] elucidated the structure of naturally occurring luteinizing hormone releasing hormone (LHRH). Since then, numerous synthetic analogs have been developed by substitution of a D-amino acid at the sixth position along the decapeptide chain and alteration of the N-terminus by substitution of an ethylamide moiety for glycine. These modifications create compounds with greatly enhanced potency compared to naturally occurring LHRH because of increased receptor affinity and reduced susceptibility to enzymatic degradation.

The action of naturally occurring LHRH is to stimulate release of the gonadotropins LH and FSH from the anterior pituitary. In response, testosterone is released by the Leydig cells of the testis. In the physiologic setting, LHRH is released in pulses necessary for its action. Chronic administration of powerful synthetic analogs of LHRH results in a depletion of pituitary LH followed by a down regulation of LHRH receptors. As a result, the pituitary becomes refractory or insensitive to further LHRH stimulation (Fig 8–4). The subsequent gonadotropin suppression and reduction in serum testosterone levels have predicated the use of LHRH analogs in patients with prostatic cancer.

Administration of synthetic LHRH anologs initially results in the stimulation of LH and FSH and, consequently, testosterone. Peak levels may reach 150% to 170% of basal levels by the third or fourth day of treatment.[14] Subsequently, there is a rapid and profound suppression of the gonadotropins and testosterone. By two weeks, serum testosterone is below basal levels, and castrate levels

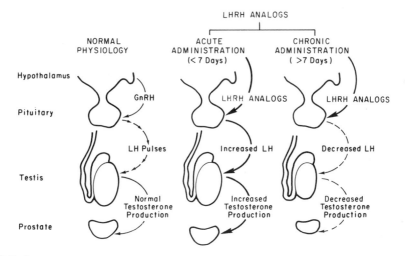

FIG 8–4.
Schematic diagram of endocrine effects of LHRH analogs. Initially serum testosterone level is increased. With long-term administration, suppression of pituitary gonadotropins occurs, producing castrate levels of serum testosterone.

are attained by one month of continuous therapy (Fig 8–5). There has been no evidence of an "escape" phenomenon in patients receiving long-term LHRH therapy at adequate doses[15] (Fig 8–6).

Numerous synthetic analogs of LHRH have been developed but the in vivo action of each appears to be similar. Therefore, production of the desired

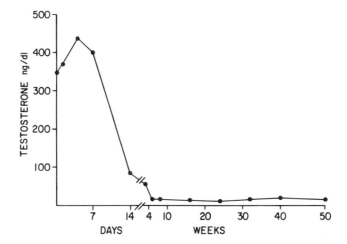

FIG 8–5.
Typical changes in serum testosterone level after initiation of daily subcutaneous therapy with an LHRH analog. Elevation of testosterone above basal levels occurs during the first week of therapy followed by rapid, profound suppression. By one month, castrate levels have been obtained in all patients.

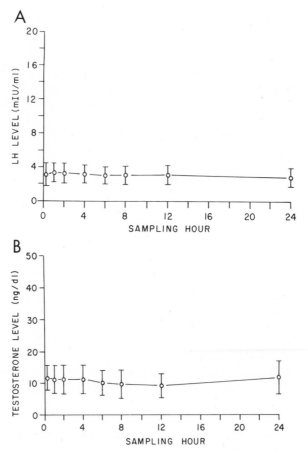

FIG 8–6.

A, LH levels determined at multiple times throughout the day in patients receiving LHRH analog therapy (leuprolide, 1 mg subcutaneously daily) for at least one year. No stimulation above basal, suppressed levels is evident. **B,** testosterone values from the same group of patients. No elevation is seen, and castrate levels have been maintained in all patients.

endocrine effect is dependent upon adequate doses and route of administration. Since LHRH analogs are proteins, parenteral administration is required. Intranasal inhalation is possible, but most clinical studies have used subcutaneous administration. Currently, one analog, leuprolide, has been approved by the U.S. Food and Drug Administration for treatment of patients with prostatic cancer. The recommended daily dose is 1 mg, administered as a 0.2-ml subcutaneous injection. Depo formulations of LHRH analogs are undergoing clinical testing.

Numerous clinical studies using LHRH analogs in men with prostatic cancer have been conducted. Most have concluded that these compounds provide a safe, alternative form of therapy with therapeutic results equivalent to those obtained with orchiectomy or estrogen administration.[16–18] The largest randomized study was conducted by the Leuprolide Study Group and showed a similar therapeutic response between patients treated with 1 mg of leuprolide daily and those receiving 3 mg of oral DES daily.[19]

LHRH analogs generally have been well tolerated and free of major side effects. Gynecomastia does not occur, and there is no apparent drug-related increase in thromboembolic complications or cardiovascular deaths. Most patients develop vasomotor hot flashes, which can be quite troublesome on occasions. Ergotamine-containing compounds may decrease the severity of hot flashes.

Because of the initial rise in the serum testosterone level that occurs with LHRH therapy, there is at least a potential for disease "flare" or exacerbation of disease-related symptoms during the first week of treatment. Some 10% to 15% of patients with bone pain prior to therapy report an increase in severity of pain during the first week of treatment. By one month, there is no apparent difference in pain response between patients treated with an LHRH analog and those receiving alternative hormonal therapy. Most patients do not develop any adverse signs or symptoms because of the initial testosterone elevation. Nevertheless, certain patients probably should be excluded from receiving LHRH analogs as initial treatment of prostatic cancer. Included in this group would be patients with impending neurologic compromise or life-threatening metastatic disease. Azotemia secondary to ureteral obstruction may be slower to resolve than after an orchiectomy and may increase during the first two weeks of treatment.

Antiandrogens

Although a number of drugs may be included in the category of antiandrogens, the mechanism of action of each is varied and may be more complex than simple blockade of androgenic effects. However, each of these compounds has the capability of inhibiting the cellular metabolism of circulating androgen.

Megestrol Acetate

Megestrol acetate (Megace) is a synthetic steroid used for the palliative treatment of metastatic breast cancer. Megace has multiple hormonal effects similar to naturally occurring progestins, including suppression of serum testosterone levels by inhibition of pituitary gonadotropin release. In addition, megace has been shown to decrease prostatic dihydrotestosterone concentrations by competing for cytosol receptors and by blocking 5-alpha reductase.[20] The primary disadvantage of megace in the treatment of prostatic cancer is that an "escape" of testosterone suppression occurs from two to six months after the initiation of therapy. Testosterone levels rise to a near normal range after around six months of treatment although the androgen block at the cellular level may continue for a period of time after the testosterone rise. Low-dose oral estrogens are given in combination with megace to prevent the testosterone rise. If concomitant estrogens are used, clinical results with megace have apparently been equal to those obtained with alternative hormonal therapy.

Cyproterone Acetate

Cyproterone acetate is a synthetic steroid with minimal androgenic or adrenal cortical activity but pronounced progestational and antiandrogenic properties. Although cyproterone acetate is not currently approved for use in the United States, it is marketed for treatment of prostatic cancer in Europe. The drug inhibits testosterone secretion from the Leydig cells of the testis. However, the principal action occurs at a cellular level where the drug inhibits cytosolic dihydrotestosterone binding and formation of the nuclear chromatin-DHT receptor complex. The drug may be administered orally, but absorption may be incomplete with encapsulated preparations.[21]

Cyproterone acetate has been a relatively safe drug that produces clinical results equal to those obtained by orchiectomy or estrogens.[22, 23] Gynecomastia is seen in some patients, but nausea and vomiting are unusual. Apparent drug-related cardiovascular toxic reactions have been reported in one study.[23]

Ketoconazole

Ketoconazole is an orally administered synthetic imidazole derivative that is widely used in the treatment of fungal diseases. High doses of the drug block the synthesis of testosterone in the testes and adrenal glands. Testosterone synthesis in the Leydig cells is blocked at a cytochrome P-50 dependent step. This blockade and its resulting depression of serum testosterone concentration, which is observed two to eight hours after drug injection, is readily reversible and dose dependent. Doses of ketoconazole used for its antifungal effect (200 mg daily) do not cause clinical problems suggestive of androgen deficiency in most patients. However, high doses of ketoconazole given on a more frequent dosing scheme can produce a significant and steady suppression of androgen production.

The ability of ketoconazole to suppress both adrenal and testicular testosterone production has been mentioned as a possible means for improved responses in prostatic cancer patients compared to conventional hormonal treatment. Clinical data are quite preliminary.[24, 25] However, side effects may occur at the increased dose levels. Nausea and vomiting have been reported and drug-related liver toxicity has been seen in some patients.

Flutamide

Flutamide is an investigational, nonsteroidal substituted anilide devoid of androgenic, antiestrogenic, or adrenal-cortical activity.[26] The exact mechanism of action remains poorly defined, but most evidence suggests that the drug inhibits the uptake of testosterone or the binding of testosterone or dihydrotestosterone to the nuclear receptor. Thereby, the biologic effects of androgens on the secondary sex structures are prevented. Since the feedback inhibition of testosterone upon the pituitary gonadal axis may be lost, patients taking flutamide maintain normal or, perhaps, elevated levels of serum testosterone. Clinical studies comparing flutamide to alternative hormonal therapy are incomplete. The drug has been used in combination with other agents to provide suppression of both testicular and adrenal androgenic sources (See section on total androgen suppression).

In general, flutamide therapy has been well tolerated by patients. Most develop gynecomastia and breast tenderness, although this appears to be less than after estrogen therapy. Nausea and vomiting have been seen in some patients, and liver function abnormalities have also been reported. Since serum testosterone levels are not diminished, it appears that some patients are able to maintain their libido and sexual potency after flutamide treatment.[27] Randomizing studies comparing flutamide to conventional hormonal therapy as initial treatment of prostatic cancer are incomplete.

Total Androgen Suppression

Often, combinations of hormonal therapy have been used in an attempt to improve response rates or to provide palliation in patients relapsing after an initial endocrine response. Combining estrogens and orchiectomy either initially or sequentially generally has been unsuccessful. Each treatment method produces its effect by decreasing serum testosterone levels, and combination treatment simply reproduces the hormonal effects of each treatment used singly. However, orchiectomy has produced responses in some patients whose serum testosterone level had been incompletely suppressed because of poor compliance with estrogen therapy or inadequate drug doses. Similarly, LHRH analogs exert their primary effect through a decrease in serum testosterone. LHRH analog treatment of patients in relapse after an initial remission with orchiectomy or estrogens has been relatively unproductive. Likewise, few responses to orchiectomy have been seen after patients have experienced failure of LHRH treatment (Fig 8–7).

Theoretically, more sound is a treatment approach that attempts to eliminate alternative sources of androgen production, i.e., the adrenal glands. Although the substantial majority of circulating androgens are of testicular origin, there is some experimental data to support the concept that adrenal androgens may contribute to the growth of prostatic cancer. Relatively low levels of circulating androgens may be associated with intracellular dihydrotestosterone concentrations that could stimulate prostatic tumor growth.[28] Ablation of adrenal androgen production generally has been unsuccessful as treatment of patients who have relapsed after previous hormonal therapy. However, the availability of new drugs or combinations of agents capable of suppressing the effects of both testicular and adrenal androgen has prompted renewed interest in the subject of total androgen ablation in the treatment of prostatic cancer.

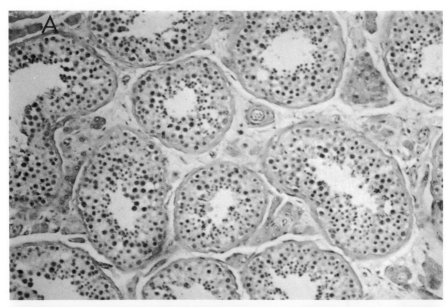

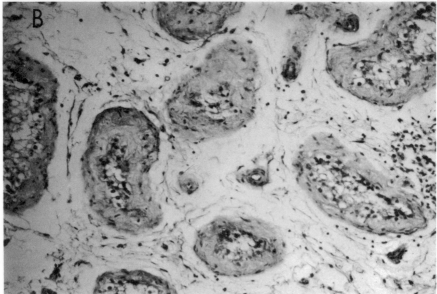

FIG 8–7.
A, histologic appearance of the testis from an orchiectomy specimen in a 63-year-old man with no prior hormonal therapy. **B,** orchiectomy specimen from a 64-year-old man who had been receiving LHRH analog therapy for one year. Marked peritubules thickening and fibrosis is evident. Few responses are observed with secondary endocrine treatment.

Adrenalectomy

Surgical.—Huggins and Scott[29] initially reported adrenalectomy for patients with prostatic cancer based on the concept that adrenal androgen ablation may be beneficial in patients relapsing after primary hormonal therapy.[29] However, in a literature review, Brendler[30] reported a 73% subjective improvement after adrenalectomy and only a 6% objective response. Most responses were of short duration. Bilateral surgical removal of the adrenal gland is a formidable surgical procedure that currently is not recommended for patients with prostatic cancer.

Medical.—Aminoglutethimide produces a medical blockade of adrenal cortical function by inhibiting the side chain cleavage of cholesterol and subsequent hydroxylation, an early step in steroidogenesis. Consequently, the synthesis of androgens, cortisols, and aldosterone is interrupted. Robinson and Thomas[31] reported a suppression of plasma testosterone to less than 10 ng/dl in a series of patients previously receiving estrogen therapy who were treated with aminoglutethimide and steroid replacement.

Side effects of aminoglutethimide treatment can be substantial, and some patients are unable to tolerate therapy. Hypotension, nausea, and vomiting may occur, and the majority of patients experience some degree of lassitude, anorexia, and depression. Nevertheless, the reported series suggest a favorable response in approximately one third of the patients, although the contribution of concomitantly administered steroids to these results is uncertain.

Hypophysectomy

Pituitary ablation via surgery, cryodestruction, or interstitial irradiation has been used primarily in patients who fail to respond or relapse after conventional hormonal therapy for prostatic cancer. In most reports, subjective pain improvement is seen in the majority of patients, but well-documented objective responses are rare.[32, 33]

The mechanism by which hypophysectomy may benefit patients with prostatic cancer in whom previous hormonal treatment has failed is uncertain. Initial interest was based upon the hypothesis of pituitary gonadotropin suppression and adrenal suppression resulting from pituitary ACTH deprivation. Hypophysectomy is known to alter levels of endorphins and enkephalins, endogenous opiate peptides that affect subjective pain interpretation and may serve as neurotransmitters in pain-modifying pathways. Since the primary response to hypophysectomy in prostatic cancer patients seems to be subjective improvement in bone pain, the effects of pituitary ablation may be related to alterations in pain perception rather than a favorable impact upon the disease process itself.

LHRH Analogs Plus Antiandrogens

The most widely publicized form of androgen ablation as first-line therapy for prostatic cancer has been the combination of an LHRH analog and an antiandrogen. Total androgen suppression theoretically can be achieved by excluding all sources of androgen production or by blocking all androgenic effects at the target cell level. In addition to surgical or medical adrenal ablation, pure antiandrogens theoretically eliminate all androgenic effects at the cellular level. However, the physiologic or slightly elevated levels of circulating testosterone that are maintained with some antiandrogens have logically led to efforts to reduce circulating testosterone as well as block the peripheral effects.

Labrie and co-workers[34] have published results suggesting that objective response rates of greater than 90% may be seen in patients receiving a combination of LHRH analog and an antiandrogen. However, criteria for determination of a true objective response are not well documented in these patients. In addition, the objective response rate of 86% for patients treated with leuprolide alone that has been reported suggests that the addition of an antiandrogen has had little if any impact.[19] Historical data have shown little response to surgical adrenal ablation after patients have failed orchiectomy. Despite some enthusiastic but poorly controlled reports to the contrary,[35] similar results have been seen in most patients treated with an antiandrogen who were in relapse after treatment with conventional hormonal therapy. Sogani and associates[36] reported results in 26 patients with prostatic cancer refractory to conventional hormonal therapy who were treated with flutamide. Six patients had evidence of a response by the criteria used, but the duration was short. McFarlane and Tolley[37] found that 12 of 14 patients failing conventional hormonal treatment had no evidence of a response to flutamide.

Considerable interest has been generated recently over the promise of improved results using an LHRH analog and an antiandrogen. Historical evidence suggests that this combination therapy is unlikely to produce improved results, but enthusiastic reports continue to emerge from current uncontrolled series. A national, multicenter study has completed accrual of over 600 patients randomized to receive either an LHRH analog plus placebo or an LHRH analog plus an antiandrogen as initial treatment of metastatic prostatic cancer. The results of this study should be most revealing and allow a scientific answer to the question of the effectiveness of total androgen ablation compared to suppression of testicular testosterone production alone.

SUMMARY AND SUGGESTIONS FOR PATIENT MANAGEMENT

Many questions regarding the ultimate effects of hormonal therapy, the optimal timing of institution of treatment, and the most effective form of therapy remain. However, the favorable response to adequate hormonal treatment in most patients with prostatic cancer is well recognized and documented. Therefore, hormonal manipulation maintains a cardinal role in the treatment of prostatic cancer.

No survival benefit has been demonstrated for patients receiving early hormonal therapy compared to those treated when symptomatic metastases are present. Overall, then, it seems reasonable and consistent with current thinking to institute hormonal treatment at a time when disease progression is evident or symptoms related to prostatic cancer occur. It is not mandatory that distant metastatic disease be evident since hormonal treatment can significantly palliate local symptoms such as recurrent bladder outlet obstruction or ureteral obstruction. When metastatic disease is newly discovered, hormonal treatment can be withheld until symptoms develop, although the interval between progression to metastatic disease and the development of symptoms usually is short. Institution of hormonal therapy earlier in the course of disease, such as at the time of discovery of pelvic lymph node metastases, is likely to prolong the time interval until metastatic disease develops but seemingly imparts no survival benefit.

For patients who will accept orchiectomy, there seems little reason to pursue treatment with any of the alternative forms of endocrine therapy. Currently, there are no convincing data that any form of endocrine therapy is more effective than orchiectomy including the methods of total androgen ablation. Oral administration of diethylstilbestrol remains the most commonly used alternative form of treatment to orchiectomy. However, because of the thromboembolic complications associated with estrogens, an LHRH analog may be an attractive alternative form of treatment, especially in patients with a history of cardiovascular disease. Antiandrogens have been studied in numerous small clinical trials, but response rates appear to be similar to those obtained with orchiectomy, estrogens, or LHRH analogs. Flutamide may offer some advantages in that some patients may maintain libido and sexual potency during treatment, but large clinical studies of this agent are incomplete.

After patients have failed an adequate initial form of endocrine therapy, durable objective or subjective responses to subsequent endocrine manipulation are unusual. Relatively nontoxic forms of treatment that suppress adrenal androgen production are being explored. However, the final results of investigations comparing methods of total androgen suppression to conventional hormonal treatment are not yet available, and early results suggest no advantage for combination therapy producing total androgen suppression.

REFERENCES

1. Huggins C, Hodges CV: Studies on prostatic cancer: I. The effect of castration, estrogen, and androgen injections on serum phosphatases in metastatic carcinoma of the prostate. *Cancer Res* 1941; 1:293.
2. Blackard CE: The Veteran's Administration Cooperative Urological Research Group studies of carcinoma of the prostate: A review. *Cancer Chemother Rep* 1975; 59:225–227.
3. Isaacs JT: New Principles in the management of metastatic prostatic cancer, in: Schroeder FH, and Richards B (eds): *Therapeutic Principles in Metastatic Prostatic Cancer*. New York, Alan R Liss, 1985.

4. Labrie F, Dupont A, Belanger A, et al: New hormonal therapy in prostatic cancer: Combined use of a pure antiandrogen and an LHRH agonist. *Hormone Res* 1983; 18:18.

5. Vest SA, Frazier TH: Survival following castration for prostatic cancer. *J Urol* 1946; 56:97–111.

6. Nesbit RM, Plumb PT: Prostatic carcinoma: A follow-up on 795 patients treated prior to endocrine era and a comparison of survival rates between these and patients treated by endocrine therapy. *Surgery* 1946; 20:263–272.

7. Nesbit RM, Baum WC: Endocrine control of prostatic carcinoma: Clinical and statistical survey of 1818 cases. *JAMA* 1950; 143:1317–1320.

8. Byar DP: The VACURG studies of cancer of the prostate. *Cancer* 1973; 32:1126–1130.

9. Blackard CE: The Veterans Administration Cooperative Urological Research Group Studies of carcinoma of the prostate: A review. *Cancer Chemother Rep* 1975; 59:225–227.

10. Maatman TJ, Gutpa MK, Montie JE: Effectiveness of castration versus intravenous estrogen therapy in producing rapid endocrine control of metastatic cancer of the prostate. *J Urol* 1985; 133:620–621. ·

11. Yanihara T, Troen P: Studies of the human testes: III. Effect of estrogen on testosterone formation in human testes in vitro. *J Clin Endocrinol* 1972; 34:968.

12. Robinson MRG, Thomas BS: Effect of hormonal therapy on plasma testosterone levels in prostatic carcinoma. *Br Med J* 1971; 4:391–394.

13. Schally AV, et al: Isolation and properties of FSH and LH releasing hormone. *Biochem Biophys Res Comm* 1971; 43:393.

14. Warner W, et al: Effect of mega-dose D-Leu-6 GnRh on the hypothalamic pituitary testicular axis as treatment of prostatic cancer. *J Clin Invest* 1983; 71:1842.

15. Smith JA Jr, for the Leuprolide Study Group: Clinical effects of gonadotropin releasing hormone analogue in metastatic carcinoma of prostate. *Urology* 1985; 25:106–114.

16. Smith JA Jr: Androgen suppression by a gonadotropin releasing hormone analog in patients with metastatic carcinoma of the prostate. *J Urol* 1984; 131:1110.

17. Wenderoth UK, Jacobi GH: Gonadotropin releasing hormone analogues for palliation of carcinoma of the prostate. *World J Urol* 1983; 1:40–48.

18. Waxman JH, et al: Treatment of advanced prostatic cancer with buserelin, an analogue of gonadotropin releasing hormone. *Br J Urol* 1983; 55:737.

19. Garnick MB, Glode LM, Smith JA Jr, for the Leuprolide Study Group: Leuprolide versus diethylstilbestrol for metastatic prostate cancer. *N Engl J Med* 1985; 311:1281–1286.

20. Geller J, Albert J, Geller S, et al: Effect of megestrol acetate (megace) in steroid metabolism and steroid binding protein in the human prostate. *J Clin Endocrine Metab* 1976; 43:1000.

21. Speck U, Jentsch D, Kuhne G, et al: Bioavailability and pharmacokinetics of 14C-cyproterone acetate after administration as a 50-mg tablet. *Drug Res* 1976; 26:1717–1720.

22. Tveter KJ, Otnes B, Hannestad R: Treatment of prostatic carcinoma with cyproterone acetate. *Scand J Urol Nephrol* 1978; 12:115–118.

23. Pavone-Macaluso, M, de Voogt HJ, Viggiano J, et al: Comparison of DES, cyproterone acetate and medroxyprogesterone acetate in the treatment of advanced prostatic cancer. *J Urol* 1986; 136:624–631.

24. Denis L, Chaban M, Mahler C: Clinical applications of ketoconazole in prostatic cancer, in Schroeder FH, Richards B (eds): *Therapeutic Principles in Metastatic Prostatic Cancer.* New York, Alan R Liss, 1985, p 319.

25. Trachtenberg J: Endocrine therapy: Non-estrogenic pharmacological manipulation. *Semin Urol* 1984; 1:288–290

26. Neri RO, Florance K, Koziol P, et al: A biologic profile of a nonsteroidal antiandrogen. Sch. 13521. *Endocrinology* 1972; 94:427–437.

27. Sogani PC, Whitmore WF Jr: Experience with flutamide in previously untreated patients with advanced prostatic cancer. *J Urol* 1979; 122:640–643.

28. Geller J, Albert J, Loza D, et al: DHT concentrations in human prostate cancer tissue. *J Clin Endocrinol Metabol* 1978; 46:440–444.

29. Huggins C, Scott WW: Bilateral adrenalectomy in prostatic cancer: Clinical features and urinary excretion of 17-ketosteroids and estrogens. *Ann Surg* 1945; 122:1031–1041.

30. Brendler H: Adrenalectomy and hypophysectomy for prostatic cancer. *Urology* 1973; 2:99–101.

31. Robinson MRG, Thomas BS: Effect of hormonal therapy on plasma testosterone levels in prostatic carcinoma. *Br Med J* 1971; 4:391–394.

32. Tindall GE, Payne NS, Nixon DW: Transsphenoidal hypophysectomy for disseminated carcinoma of the prostate gland. *J Neurosurg* 1979; 50:275.

33. Smith JA Jr, Eyre HJ, Roberts TS, et al: Transsphenoidal hypophysectomy in the management of carcinoma of the prostate. *Cancer* 1984; 53:2385.

34. Labrie F, Dupont A, Lacourciere Y, et al: Combined treatment with flutamide in association with medical or surgical castration. *J Urol* 1986; 135:71A.

35. Schroeder FH: Total androgen suppression in the management of prostatic cancer: A critical review, in Schroeder FH, Richards B (eds): *Therapeutic Principles in Metastatic Prostatic Cancer.* New York, Alan R Liss, 1985, p 307.

36. Sogani PC, Ray B, Whitmore WF Jr: Advanced prostatic carcinoma: Flutamide therapy after conventional endocrine treatment. *Urology* 1975; 6:164–166.

37. Mac Farlane JA, Tolley DA: Flutamide therapy for advanced prostatic cancer: A phase III study. *Br J Urol* 1985; 57:172–174.

9

Chemotherapy

Several factors have inhibited the use of cytotoxic chemotherapy in the treatment of patients with metastatic prostatic cancer. The advanced age of most men with prostatic cancer to some degree decreases patient tolerance to the side effects of chemotherapy. Moreover, the anticipated response to hormonal treatment has dampened enthusiasm for more toxic methods of therapy in patients with newly diagnosed metastatic disease. Patients in relapse after hormonal treatment frequently have large tumor burdens and are too ill to tolerate chemotherapy. Finally, difficulties in assessing treatment response have led to confusion regarding whether patients derive any substantial benefit from treatment.

Despite these limitations, there are increasing numbers of clinical trials using cytotoxic agents both as adjunctive treatment and as primary therapy in patients with prostatic cancer. Outside of established clinical protocols, chemotherapy is used frequently by some clinicians, primarily because of the absence of effective alternative therapy in hormone-unresponsive disease. Therefore, in order to make informed clinical decisions regarding the use of chemotherapy in prostatic cancer patients, it is appropriate to review both the results of previous studies as well as the methods of disease assessment.

DISEASE RESPONSE

The primary aims of chemotherapeutic treatment of cancer should be symptomatic improvement and prolonged patient survival. The former is primarily a subjective interpretation that may be influenced by multiple other factors. Demonstration of prolonged patient survival requires comparison to a group of "control" patients not receiving therapy. This is of particular importance in prostatic cancer, wherein the variable natural history of the disease may make treatment effects on survival difficult to determine.

Because of these difficulties, most clinical oncologic studies of the effects of chemotherapy on solid tumors have relied on objective measurements of tumor size to indicate treatment response. In general, this requires bidimensionally measurable disease that can be assessed objectively. Since most patients with metastatic prostatic cancer do not have lung or other easily measured soft-tissue metastases, determination of response is even more difficult. Trials that have been restricted to patients with classically measurable disease often have had insufficient patient numbers.

Previously, it has been suggested that patients with measurable soft-tissue metastases have a prognosis that differs (usually worse) from that of patients with bone disease only. More recently this has been questioned, and response rates and patient survival when adjusted for tumor burden are probably similar between the two groups. At any rate, it is evident that large-scale clinical trials evaluating patients with metastatic prostatic cancer must include the typical patients with bone disease only who may not have demonstrable or measurable soft-tissue metastases.

Whether bone disease alone should be considered measurable or simply evaluable has been a point of much discussion. Various methods of evaluation of response based on serial bone roentgenograms or radioisotope bone scans have emerged (Table 9–1). The relative insensitivity of bone roentgenograms compared to bone scans has led to adoption of the latter as the preferred method for evaluation of disease status. Based on their extensive studies, the National Prostatic Cancer Project (NPCP) accepted a set of criteria for determining response in prostatic cancer patients.[1] By NPCP criteria, an overall decrease of more than 50% in the volume and intensity of skeletal metastases, if accompanied by other criteria, is considered a partial response. On the other hand, any new lesion on bone scan is evidence of progressive disease. An often mentioned, but relatively rare, source of error using these definitions is that recalcification of osteolytic lesions may mimic enlarging osteoblastic areas and be interpreted as disease progression in some responding patients.

Another important variable besides bone scan used to assess treatment response in patients is acid phosphatase. Although a useful tumor marker, the level of acid phosphatase does not necessarily correlate with tumor response. Some 20% or 25% of patients with demonstrable metastatic disease have nor-

TABLE 9–1.
Criteria for Partial Response Among Selected Cooperative Groups

	TUMOR MASS	ACID PHOSPHATASE	LYTIC BONE	PERFORMANCE STATUS
National Prostatic Cancer Project	50% decrease	Return to normal	Recalcification	No decrease
Southwest Oncology Group	50% decrease	50% decrease	Not a criterion	No decrease
Uro-Oncology Group	50% decrease	Return to normal	Recalcification	No decrease
Eastern Cooperative Oncology Group	50% decrease	50% decrease	Not a criterion	Not a criterion

mal serum acid phosphatase levels. The degree of elevation of serum acid phosphatase has not been shown to be a prognostic factor independent of tumor burden.

In addition to problems in determining the significance of initial acid phosphatase levels, variable interpretations regarding changes in acid phosphatase during therapy exist. Diurnal or, perhaps, sporadic variations in acid phosphatase levels occur. In some studies, a 50% decrease in acid phosphatase concentrations is considered to be indicative of a response. By other criteria, including the NPCP, acid phosphatase must decrease to normal levels to be considered significant.[2] At the other end of the spectrum, elevation of the serum acid phosphatase level during treatment is considered disease progression by some groups, while acid phosphatase elevation alone does not constitute progression by the NPCP criteria.[3]

A final consideration of paramount importance in assessing response rate in previous chemotherapeutic studies is inclusion of the "stable" category as a favorable response. Many patients, including some with an obvious, durable clinical response to hormonal therapy, do not show objective improvement on bone scan. Furthermore, it has been argued that patients with disease progression prior to treatment who exhibit stable disease on a bone scan have demonstrated a legitimate response.[4] An alternative explanation, however, is that stable disease is simply an observation of the prolonged natural history of the disease in some patients. In addition, Yagoda and others[5] have pointed out that many patients have not had clearly progressive disease prior to study entry on some protocols. Although the NPCP has shown that patients with stable disease have a survival duration similar to those with a partial response, prolonged survival compared with untreated controls has not been demonstrated.

CYTOTOXIC AGENTS

The multiple factors discussed above introduce many variables into the interpretation of disease response to various chemotherapeutic regimens. What follows is a review of selected agents in which at least some activity has been suggested or demonstrated in prostatic cancer. A more comprehensive list of agents is shown in Table 9–2.

Cyclophosphamide (Cytoxan)

Cyclophosphamide (Cytoxan) is one of the most extensively studied and frequently used chemotherapeutic drugs for treatment of prostatic cancer. The drug is an alkylating agent that produces cross-linkage of adjacent DNA strands. As with other chemotherapy, documented complete or partial responses are unusual. Disease stabilization, considered a response by some groups, may be seen in about one third of patients. The NPCP has studied Cytoxan at a dose of 1,000 mg/sq m intravenously every three weeks.[6] Only 5% of patients had

TABLE 9–2.

Objective Response Rates for Selected Single Agents and Combinations in
Prostatic Cancer*

AGENTS	OBJECTIVE REGRESSION (COMPLETE OR PARTIAL RESPONSE)	STABILIZATION†
Cyclophosphamide	5%	25%–50%
Doxorubicin	4%–27%	25%–60%
Cis-platinum	4%–29%	10%–30%
5-Fluorouracil	5%–20%	10%–35%
Cyclophosphamide plus Adriamycin	0%–25%	15%–30%
Adriamycin, mitomycin-C, 5-fluorouracil	50%	. . .
Cyclophosphamide, methotrexate, 5-fluorouracil	10%–15%	20%–45%

*Various response criteria used among different studies.
†Considered a "response" by some groups.

objective tumor regression. If disease stabilization was included, cytoxan was
thought to be more effective than standard palliative therapy without cytotoxic
agents.

Doxorubicin (Adriamycin)

Doxorubicin has also been studied as a single agent in patients with metastatic prostatic cancer. Yagoda[7] studied doses of Adriamycin at 30, 45, and 60
mg/sq m intravenously every three weeks but found objective response in only
two of 46 patients treated. Using various definitions of response, partial regression has been seen in 15% to 27% of patients reported in other studies although the median response duration has only been around three months and
overall patient survival usually only six to nine months.[8]

Cis-Diamminedichloroplatinum

Cis-platinum has effects similar to an alkylating agent and produces cross-
linking on adjacent strands of DNA. Merrin and Beckley[9] reported a partial
objective response in 29% of patients with metastatic prostatic cancer using a
regimen consisting of 1 mg/kg IV of cis-platinum weekly for six weeks and
then every three weeks thereafter. However, Yagoda and colleagues[5] found
partial response in only 12% of patients using 50 to 70 mg/sq m of IV cis-
platinum every three weeks. The NPCP project studied cis-platinum in patients
who had not received previous irradiation and used a dose of 60 mg/sq m IV
on days 1, 4, 21, and 24 followed by monthly doses thereafter. Objective
regression was seen in only 4% of patients, but stable disease (considered a
response) was seen in 32%. The median duration of response and survival was
only four months.[10]

Combination Chemotherapy

In addition to single-agent trials, numerous multiagent chemotherapy trials have been conducted.[1, 11, 12] Considering the low response rates seen with any of these studies, it is difficult to demonstrate definitive superiority of combination therapy over single agents. However, an objective response rate of 50% was reported for patients receiving the three-drug combination of Adriamycin (50 mg/sq m on day 1), mitomycin-C (10 mg/sq m on day 1) and 5-fluorouracil (750 mg/sq m on days 1 and 2).[13] Treatments were repeated every three weeks as long as patients could tolerate therapy. Recalcification of lytic bone lesions or decrease in number of blastic metastases on bone scan were considered treatment responses if at least a 50% reduction in the serum acid phosphatase level also occurred. Toxicity of this regimen is considerable, and two of the first 42 patients treated died of myelosuppression. The average response duration has been approximately seven months, but improvement in survival compared with untreated patients has not been demonstrated. Many patients tolerate this regimen poorly, but the reported response rates of this regimen appear to be superior to those obtained with single-agent chemotherapy. However, preliminary results of a Southwest Oncology Group study have not confirmed objective responses this high using the same regimen.

Estramustine Phosphate (Emcyt)

Emcyt is a synthetic combination of nitrogen mustard and estradiol. The drug is reported to bind to the estrogen receptors in prostatic cancer cells or to an intracellular binding protein. The alkylating effect of the nitrogen mustard is then activated by acid phosphatases.[14] There has been considerable question whether the sole effects of the drug are due to the endocrine effects of the estrogen. In previously untreated patients, pituitary luteinizing hormone secretion is suppressed as well as serum testosterone levels. Accordingly, high response rates are observed in patients who have not received previous endocrine therapy. In some studies, it has been suggested that the initial response rate in Emcyt-treated patients exceeds that of alternative hormonal therapy, although this has not been verified in other studies. In patients who have relapsed after previous hormonal therapy, objective response rates have been seen in up to 35% of patients.[15] However, partial regression was seen in only 6% of patients with hormonally refractory tumor in the NPCP study of estramustine as a single agent when 600 mg/sq m was administered orally on a daily basis.[16] In other NPCP studies, Emcyt has demonstrated no superiority over cis-platinum[17] or methotrexate,[10] and the mean duration of survival in treated patients was about ten months.

Approximately 20% of Emcyt-treated patients experience nausea and vomiting, and 15% have been reported to have abnormalities of liver function test results.[18] Therefore, in the absence of consistently demonstrated superiority of Emcyt over standard methods of hormonal therapy, most clinicians have had little enthusiasm for the use of Emcyt as the initial treatment in patients with metastatic prostatic cancer. In hormonally refractory patients, objective responses are minimal and there is no demonstrated improvement in patient survival.

EARLY INSTITUTION OF CHEMOTHERAPY

Most clinical trials of prostatic cancer have been conducted in patients with hormone-refractory disease and large tumor burden. Therefore, it has been suggested that this may account for the overall poor responses and that improved results could be obtained with earlier initiation of chemotherapy. Some studies have evaluated the combination of hormonal therapy plus cytotoxic chemotherapy in patients with newly diagnosed metastatic disease. The NPCP found no difference in response between patients randomized to receive either standard hormonal therapy consisting of DES (3 mg daily) or orchiectomy compared to those receiving DES plus Cytoxan at 1 gm/sq m or Emcyt (600 mg/sq m orally daily) plus Cytoxan. Median response and duration of survival were similar among all three treatment arms.[3] Merrin[19] treated 34 patients with orchiectomy, 1 mg of DES daily, and cis-platinum (1 mg/kg weekly for six weeks and then every three weeks thereafter). Partial responses were observed in 65% of patients and stable disease in 32%. These response rates are not unlike those that could be achieved with endocrine treatment alone, and the mean duration of response was only nine months.

Only minimal information is available regarding the value of early institution of chemotherapy in patients with stage D1 tumors (positive pelvic lymph nodes in the absence of distant disease). DeVere White and associates[20] used adjuvant chemotherapy consisting of Cytoxan, 750 mg/sq m, and Adriamycin, 50 mg/sq m, and found disease progression in 33% of patients who received adjunctive chemotherapy compared to 48% who did not, but duration of follow-up was limited.

Randomized, prospective trials to evaluate the value of early chemotherapy either in an adjunctive fashion or in newly diagnosed metastatic disease seem warranted. However, in the absence of demonstrated prolongation of patient survival using chemotherapy, and considering the known toxic effects of treatment, there seems little justification for recommendation of early chemotherapy for most patients with prostatic cancer.

IMMUNOTHERAPY

Cryosurgery has been used to treat the primary tumor in patients with prostatic cancer based on the belief that antiprostatic antibodies could be induced. However, no objective evidence of an immune response after cryosurgery has been evident and objective regression of metastatic disease has been unusual.[21] Local tumor regression has been seen in up to 60% of patients, but most had received concomitant hormonal therapy. Overall, there seems no evidence of immunologic stimulation in patients treated with cryosurgery for prostatic cancer, and local control rates are inferior to those obtained with radical prostatectomy or external irradiation.

Nonspecific immunotherapy using *Bacillus* Calmette-Guerin (BCG) has been reported in patients with prostatic cancer. Guinan and colleagues[22] administered 2.3×10^8 Tice organisms every four months intradermally in prostatic cancer patients. Various stages of prostatic cancer were included and some patients had received prior hormonal therapy while others had not. Nevertheless, median survival was 38 weeks in BCG-treated patients compared with 28 weeks in patients not receiving BCG. Brosman[23] randomized 42 patients to receive eight weekly intradermal injections of 3×10^9 organisms of Tice BCG or no therapy. Previous endocrine therapy had failed in all patients, and no survival advantage was detected in the BCG-treated patients.

SUMMARY

The results of chemotherapy for prostatic cancer patients have been disappointing. Multiple factors have contributed to the difficulty in administering cytotoxic chemotherapy to these patients. Objective responses are unusual, and no survival advantage for chemotherapy-treated patients have been demonstrated. In general, then, there seems little justification for recommending chemotherapy for most patients with prostatic cancer. When used in an adjuvant setting or at the first diagnosis of metastatic disease, the toxic effects of treatment seem excessive considering the lack of demonstrated effectiveness. For hormonally refractory patients, the objective responses or symptomatic improvement seen occasionally are short lived and no survival benefit can be demonstrated.

REFERENCES

1. Schmidt JD: Chemotherapy of hormone resistant stage D prostatic cancer. *J Urol* 1980; 123:797–805.
2. Citrin DL, Cohen AI, Harbert J, et al: Systemic treatment of advanced prostate cancer: Development of a new system for defining response. *J Urol* 1981; 125:224–227.
3. Murphy GP, Beckley S, Brady MF, et al: Treatment of newly diagnosed metastatic prostate cancer patients with chemotherapy agents in combination with hormones versus hormones alone. *Cancer* 1983; 51:1264–1272.
4. Slack NH, Mittelman A, Brady MF, et al: The importance of the stable category for chemotherapy treatment patients with advanced and relapsing prostate cancer. *Cancer* 1980; 46:2393–2402.
5. Yagoda A, Watson RC, Natale RB, et al: A critical analysis of response criteria in

patients with prostate cancer treated with cis-platinum II. *Cancer* 1979; 44:1553–1562.

6. Scott WW, Gibbons RP, Johnson DE, et al: The continued evaluation of chemotherapy in patients with advanced carcinoma of the prostate. *J Urol* 1976; 116:211–213.

7. Yagoda A: Advances in chemotherapy. in Javadpour N (ed): *Recent Advances in Urologic Cancer.* Baltimore, Williams & Wilkins, 1982, pp 223–233.

8. O'Bryan RM, Baker LH, Gottlieb JE, et al: Dose response evaluation of adriamycin in human neoplasia. *Cancer* 1977; 39:1940–1948.

9. Merrin CE, Beckley S: Treatment of estrogen resistant stage D carcinoma of the prostate with cisdiammine dichloroplatinum. *Urology* 1979; 13:267–272.

10. Loening SA, Beckley S, Brady MF, et al: Comparison of estramustine phosphate, methotrexate and cis-platinum in patients with advanced, hormone refractory prostate cancer. *J Urol* 1983; 129:1001–1006.

11. Herr HW: Cyclophosphamide, methotrexate and 5 fluorouracil combination chemotherapy versus chloroethyl-cyclohexyl-nitrosourea in the treatment of metastatic prostatic cancer. *J Urol* 1982; 127:462–465.

12. Muss HB, Howard V, Richards F, et al: Cyclophosphamide versus cyclophosphamide, methotrexate and 5 fluorouracil in advanced prostatic cancer. *Cancer* 1981; 47:1949–1953.

13. Logothetis CJ, von Eschenbach AC, Samuels ML, et al: DMF regimen for hormone refractory adenocarcinoma of the prostate—the first 42 patients. *Cancer Bull* 1982; 34:26–28.

14. Nilsson T, Jonsson G: Primary treatment of prostate carcinoma with estramustine phosphate: Preliminary report. *J Urol* 1976; 115:168–169.

15. Fossa SD, Miller A: Treatment of advanced carcinoma of the prostate with estramustine phosphate. *J Urol* 1976; 115:406–408.

16. Murphy GP, Gibbons RP, Johnson DE: A comparison of estramustine phosphate and streptozotocin in patients with advanced prostatic carcinoma who have had extensive irradiation. *J Urol* 1977; 118:288–291.

17. Soloway MS, Beckley S, Brady MF: A comparison of estramustine phosphate versus cis-platinum alone versus estramustine phosphate plus cis-platinum in patients with advanced hormone refractory prostate cancer who had extensive irradiation to the pelvis or lumbosacral area. *J Urol* 1983; 129:56–61.

18. Benson RC, Wear JB, Gill GM: Treatment of stage D hormone resistant carcinoma of the prostate with estramustine phosphate. *J Urol* 1979; 121:454.

19. Merrin CE: Treatment of previously untreated (by hormonal manipulation) stage D adenocarcinoma of the prostate with combined orchiectomy, estrogen, and cis-diamminedichloro-platinum. *Urology* 1980; 15:123–126.

20. De Vere White R, Babaian RK, Krikorian J, et al: Adjuvant chemotherapy for stage D_1 adenocarcinoma of prostate. *Urology* 1983; 21:270–272.

21. Schmidt JD: Cryosurgical prostatectomy. *Cancer* 1973; 32:1141–1144.

22. Guinan P, Toronchi E, Shaw M, et al: BCG adjuvant therapy in stage D prostate cancer. *Urology* 1982; 20:401–403.

23. Brosman S: Nonspecific immunotherapy in GU cancer, in Crispen RG (ed): *Neoplasm Immunity: Solid Tumor Therapy.* Philadelphia, Franklin Institute Press, 1977, pp 97–107.

10

Management of Complications of Prostatic Cancer

One of the more challenging areas in clinical medicine is the appropriate management of the problems that can arise from local extension of tumors or metastatic cancer. In particular, this applies to prostatic cancer. Rapid disease progression is not inevitable, and complications that do arise may require long-term management. Decisions regarding how aggressively certain complications should be approached must be made in the context of the expected overall patient survival and anticipation of other problems that may become evident later.

The various problems discussed in this chapter are all ones that are encountered with some frequency in patients with prostatic cancer. It is recognized that the most important factor influencing clinical decisions in these settings is the overall condition and prognosis for an individual patient. However, the various therapeutic options discussed are those that should be considered for the palliation or more definitive control of complications arising from prostatic cancer.

BONE PAIN

Since prostatic cancer frequently metastasizes to bone, pain is often a prominent feature in metastatic disease. In prostatic cancer, metastatic bone lesions most often are blastic but also may be more lytic in nature and appearance. Various therapeutic options are available to either eliminate or control pain due to prostatic cancer bone metastases.

Endocrine Therapy

Patients with bone pain from metastatic prostatic cancer who have received no prior hormonal therapy should be treated initially with some form of endocrine manipulation (see chapter 8). Any form of hormonal therapy that adequately deprives the prostatic cancer cell of serum androgen is likely to produce a favorable symptomatic response in approximately 80% of treated patients. The symptomatic response usually commences soon after serum androgens are suppressed to the castrate range. Accordingly, a decrease in bone pain occurs most rapidly after orchiectomy since castrate levels of testosterone are achieved within 12 hours. After oral estrogen administration, testosterone is maximally suppressed within three or four days. With LHRH analogs, castrate levels of circulating androgens are not uniformly reached until after three or four weeks of drug administration. In addition, the initial elevation of testosterone that occurs after LHRH analog administration may actually result in an increase in bone pain within the first week or two of therapy in some patients.[1]

Once castrate levels of serum androgens have been obtained, the duration of symptomatic response appears to be equivalent among various forms of hormonal therapy. The mean remission duration is approximately 18 months. When relapse occurs, symptoms of bone pain often return and objective disease progression is usually evident. Mean patient survival is usually around six months with endocrine unresponsive disease.

Once adequate deprivation of serum androgens has been obtained, further endocrine manipulation usually does not have any substantial effect on bone pain. Megestrol acetate (discussed in chapter 8) and various antiandrogens have been added to standard hormonal therapy, but prolonged, definite symptomatic responses are unusual.[2] However, it is important to maintain testosterone suppression even in a patient with bone pain and progressive disease. Presumably, certain tumor cells maintain their androgen responsiveness and continue to be suppressed by endocrine therapy.

External Irradiation

External irradiation can be an effective form of palliation for localized areas of symptomatic bone metastases. When the area of tumor metastasis is well defined and in a region previously nonirradiated, some 60% to 70% of patients experience pain improvement or disappearance after localized irradiation.[3]

The degree and duration of pain relief achieved with external irradiation depends to some degree on the tumor size and location. Generally, about 2,000 rad of radiation is delivered in 200-rad fractions. Side effects usually are not significant and are dependent primarily upon the location of the metastases and by other tissues or organs within the radiated field. Significant pain improvement is usually noticed toward the end of the planned course of treatment but sometimes is not seen until after treatment has been completed.

Although several areas can be treated simultaneously, the diffuse nature of the skeletal metastases from prostatic cancer and the multiple sites of bone pain that may ensue are one of the primary limitations of irradiation for palliation of bone pain. Tissue tolerance and, therefore, radiation doses are limited in previously irradiated areas. Multiple treatments or treatment of large volumes of bone marrow may compound the anemia often seen in patients with metastatic prostatic cancer.

Half-Body Irradiation

In situations wherein the diffuse nature of the bone metastases and pain preclude effective therapy with localized irradiation, hemibody therapy has been used. Only modest doses of radiation to any given area are tolerated. Generally, 500 to 700 rad is delivered to the upper body, while lower-body doses are up to 1,000 rad. Nausea and vomiting occur in over half of the patients, and pneumonitis may result after treatment to the upper body half. Anemia or leukopenia can be life threatening in 10% to 15% of patients. The pain improvement experienced by patients receiving hemibody irradiation frequently is less marked than that achieved with treatment to localized, more defined areas. The Radiation Therapy Oncology Group found that 70% of patients with prostate cancer treated with hemibody irradiation achieved at least some pain relief for a median of 15 months.[4]

Hypophysectomy

Pituitary ablation via surgery, external irradiation, or interstitial irradiation has been used in patients with metastatic prostatic cancer. Although objective tumor regression and prolonged patient survival have not been demonstrated, subjective improvement in bone pain has been in some 50% to 70% of patients so treated. This has been manifested by decreased patient perception of pain and a decreased need for analgesics. Unlike breast cancer, the success of hypophysectomy performed for prostatic cancer does not depend upon the degree or duration of a previous endocrine response.[5] In fact, the demonstration that patients may obtain subjective relief in the face of obvious objective tumor progression suggests that the favorable effects of hypophysectomy that are seen may be unrelated to any endocrine effects or a favorable influence upon the tumor itself. Hypophysectomy is known to alter levels of endorphins and enkephalins, endogenous opiates that serve as neurotransmitters along pain-modifying pathways. Thus, the beneficial effects of hypophysectomy may be merely upon pain perceptive processes.

We found a subjective improvement in bone pain after transsphenoidal hypophysectomy in 73% of our patients although no objective responses were observed. The duration of pain improvement varied and ranged between three months and 24 months with a mean of nine months. Despite this, hypophysectomy seems to be only occasionally useful in patients with prostatic cancer. Alternative means of bone pain control should be exhausted first. Expected patient survival is relatively short, and it is highly questionable whether the benefit obtained from hypophysectomy warrants the morbidity, period of hospitalization, and expense of the procedure.

Etidronate Disodium

Etidronate disodium (Didronel) is a drug that inhibits bone resorption and is marketed for use in patients with Paget's disease. Since metastatic deposits of prostatic cancer cells frequently produce resorption of cortical bone,[6] it has been suggested that etidronate disodium may be useful for palliation of hormone-resistant bone pain in prostatic cancer patients. Small, nonrandomized clinical trials using sodium etidronate have suggested that the drug is efficacious in prostatic cancer patients and can produce significant palliation of bone pain.[7] In addition, other drugs that inhibit bone resorption have shown apparently favorable results.[7] A large, prospective, randomized trial comparing etidronate disodium with placebo is incomplete. However, preliminary results suggest that the drug is of limited usefulness in most prostatic cancer patients.

Steroids

In patients with end-stage prostatic cancer, it has been an observation of many clinicians that glucocorticoids can produce short-term subjective improvement. Patients generally experience an increased overall feeling of well-being, probably as a nonspecific effect of steroid administration. In addition, some bone pain relief may be observed. Whether this is due to central actions of the drug or to a decrease in the inflammation and edema that may surround metastatic bone lesions is uncertain. The improvement obtained is usually of short duration. Nevertheless, oral administration of steroids frequently is useful for short-term palliation of symptoms of end-stage prostatic cancer.

Analgesics

Despite the various measures discussed above, bone pain requiring analgesics is a prominent feature of metastatic prostatic cancer. Although methods should be used to attempt to eliminate the source of the pain, analgesics frequently are necessary and should be used to alleviate pain. The pain associated with bone metastases from prostatic cancer may be intermittent or related to specific physical activities but often is a relatively constant deep, throbbing pain.

There are no known peculiarities about the response of prostatic cancer bone pain to analgesics compared with other pains. Aspirin or nonsteroidal anti-inflammatory drugs frequently are useful for relatively mild pain, and there is evidence that nonnarcotic analgesics may be particularly effective in relieving the pain associated with bone metastasis.[8] Usually, as the tumor progresses, oral narcotics such as codeine, oxycodone, meperidine, or morphine become necessary. In some circumstances, it is preferable for patients to take narcotics on a routine basis rather than attempt to eliminate the pain when it is at its most intense level. Therefore, longer-acting oral narcotics such as methadone may be useful. The long half-life of this drug allows continued maintenance of serum drug levels that helps suppress pain. It must be remembered that re- peated frequent dosing can be cumulative and result in depression of mental function and lethargy. Maintenance doses of methadone can be supplemented as needed with shorter-acting oral narcotics.

Too often, patients with pain from metastatic cancer are undermedicated and never receive adequate pain relief. Considering the short anticipated life expectancy, drug addiction or abuse is not a concern. When increasing doses of pain medications are required, it should be remembered that an increase of, for example, codeine from 15 mg to 30 mg is a doubling of the dose. However, patients already receiving 30 mg on a routine basis may experience less pain relief by a further increase of 15 mg since this would only represent a 50% increase in the analgesic dose. Usually, adequate pain relief can be obtained with optimal doses of oral narcotics. Occasionally, it is helpful for a family member to administer intramuscular drugs to the patient if he is intol- erant of oral medication or not receiving adequate pain relief from it.

Intrathecal catheters for administration of narcotic drugs occasionally are useful. Trigger-point injections of local anesthetics may relieve localized areas of pain.[9] Neurosurgically implanted Omaya reservoirs allow intraventricular administration of narcotics, which can decrease the total dose necessary for pain relief.

Ideally, narcotics or other analgesics are titrated to a dose that adequately suppresses bone pain without significantly interfering with mental function. The most common side effect of narcotics in patients with metastatic prostatic cancer is constipation. Due to decreased bowel motility, this frequently can be a distressing and difficult problem for patients. Liberal fluid intake, stool sof- teners, bulk laxatives, and suppositories or enemas should be used. Patients should be advised of the likelihood of problems with constipation and of the various means to prevent or treat it.

SPINAL CORD COMPRESSION

One of the most devastating complications of metastatic prostatic cancer is spinal cord compression from vertebral collapse. The cervical, thoracic, and lumbar vertebrae are common sites of metastatic disease, and lower-extremity neurologic defects are seen in some 10% of these patients.[10] Symptoms of neurologic compromise such as sciatica, paresthesias, or muscle weakness sig- nal potential neurologic compromise and should lead to immediate diagnostic studies. Occasionally, a hypotonic neurogenic bladder is the initial sign of spinal cord compression from prostatic cancer.

Whenever spinal cord compression is suspected, appropriate evaluation should proceed promptly. Plain films of the spine may show vertebral collapse, although this does not necessarily correlate with spinal cord compression. Tra- ditionally, a myelogram has been used to demonstrate areas of narrowing or complete block within the spinal canal (Fig 10–1). More recently, CT scanning or magnetic resonance imaging of the spine has been used to demonstrate areas of tumor compression (Fig 10–2).

Once symptomatic compression of the spinal cord has been demonstrated, therapeutic intervention should be undertaken. The degree of functional return is directly related to the duration of compression. Bilateral orchiectomy should be performed promptly if the patient has not had prior hormonal therapy. High-dose IV steroids (100 mg of hydrocortisone) can provide some immediate improvement in edema and prevent further neurologic compromise until more definitive intervention is undertaken. It remains controversial whether external irradiation or surgical decompressive laminectomy should be

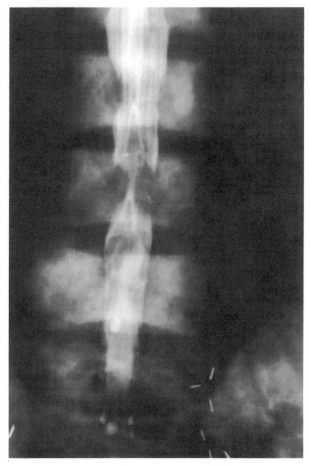

FIG 10–1.
Lumbar myelogram showing extrinsic compression of spinal cord at the L-3 vertebral body from metastatic prostatic cancer. The patient developed the acute onset of lower extremity weakness but had rapid improvement after an orchiectomy. Blastic changes in the vertebral bodies are easily seen.

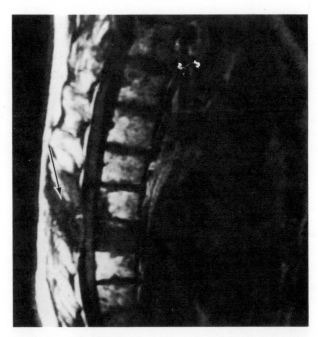

FIG 10–2.
MRI scan showing tumor involvement of T-9 vertebra with soft-tissue extension and compression of spinal cord.

undertaken as the initial treatment for patients with spinal cord compression from prostatic cancer metastases if hormonal therapy has been used previously (Fig 10–3). After external irradiation, relief of pressure on the spinal cord may not occur for several days. In fact, before that time, there may be an increase in pressure due to radiation-induced edema. Therefore, we have tended to recommend an emergency laminectomy for most patients with an acute deficit and reserved external irradiation for patients with subacute or impending problems.

Laminectomy is performed with the patient in the prone position, and pressure upon the spinal cord is relieved by removal of the overlying bone and bulk tumor mass. If the deficit is of short duration, rapid improvement in symptoms and functional recovery result. However, in patients in whom a substantial deficit has persisted for longer than 12 hours, functional return may be slow and incomplete. Prolonged periods of rehabilitation may be required.[11]

Because of the sometimes unsatisfactory result when intervention is delayed until symptomatic compression is evident, anticipation and early intervention are mandatory. If vertebral collapse is evident or if there are any signs of neurologic impairment, external irradiation should be used before the onset of muscle weakness. Occasionally, stabilizing rods are used when extensive tumor destruction has compromised the stability of the spinal column.

PATHOLOGIC FRACTURE

In addition to vertebral collapse or epidural spinal compression from prostatic cancer, tumor metastases to the long bones may result in cortical weakness and pathologic fracture. Most often, this occurs in the humerus or femur (Fig 10–4). Since most bone metastases from prostatic cancer are osteoblastic in nature, it has been suggested that they are somewhat more resistent to pathologic fracture than the osteolytic lesions seen with the other tumors. However, pathologic fracture can occur and can be a disabling problem.

Hormonal therapy should be instituted if it has not been used previously.

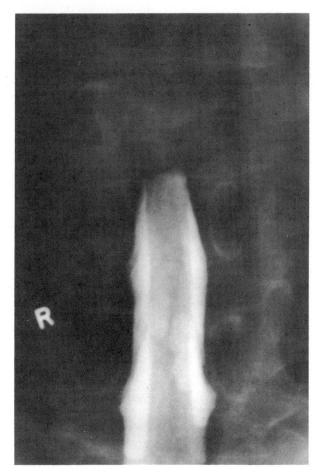

FIG 10–3.
Myelogram showing complete block of spinal column at the L3-4 interspace and a patient failing hormonal therapy. Only minimal improvement was seen after an emergency lumbar laminectomy.

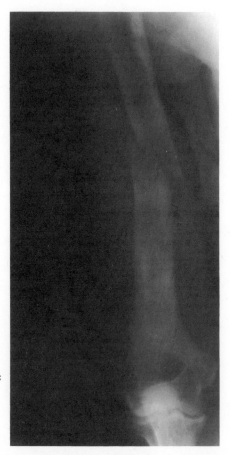

FIG 10–4.
Pathologic fracture of humerus at site of lytic
bone metastases from prostatic cancer.
Although most metastatic lesions from
prostatic cancer are blastic in nature,
pathologic fracture may occur, especially in
the humerus or femur.

In patients in whom endocrine treatment has failed, external irradiation should
be administered to symptomatic areas of metastasis in the long bones and may
be considered as a prophylactic measure in asymptomatic lesions of the femur
and humerus if they are progressing in size. Once a fracture has occurred,
spontaneous healing after immobilization usually occurs at a rate approaching
that of normal bones.[12] However, intramedullary rods may be necessary and
may significantly decrease the pain and improve the functional mobility of the
patient. After rods have been placed, external irradiation should be administered to the affected area if the radiation tolerance of the tissue has not been
exceeded.

BLADDER OUTLET OBSTRUCTION

Bladder outlet obstruction is a frequent manifestation of prostatic cancer.
The symptoms of obstruction, i.e., hesitancy, frequency, dribbling, or a slow
urinary stream, may mimic those associated with benign prostatic enlargement.

However, the symptoms may be more rapid in onset and, especially in younger men, the rapid development of urinary retention should raise a suspicion of prostatic cancer. In most patients, examination of the prostate when the patient presents for evaluation of obstructive symptoms shows induration or nodularity typical of prostatic cancer. In some patients (stage A prostatic cancer) the diagnosis is unsuspected until after prostatectomy. Management of obstructive symptoms in patients with prostatic cancer and indications for surgery may differ from those associated with benign prostatic enlargement and depend to some extent on the stage of the primary tumor.

In patients being considered for radical prostatectomy, transurethral prostatectomy should not be performed since this may increase the difficulty of the radical surgery. If a suspicious nodule is present, biopsy or aspiration should be performed without TURP. Management of obstructive symptoms in patients in whom external irradiation is planned deserves comment. Although eventual regression of prostatic size occurs in most patients after external irradiation, prostatic swelling and interstitial edema due to the acute radiation injury may exacerbate any obstructive symptoms. In addition, delayed healing of the prostatic fossa may occur if transurethral prostatecotmy is performed within several months of the completion of external irradiation. Therefore, relief of obstructive symptoms is desirable before the initiation of external beam radiation therapy. Most often, this is achieved by a transurethral prostatectomy. Radiation treatment is initiated several months later, when reepithelialization of the prostatic fossa is complete. As an alternative, hormonal therapy may be used, although the response in terms of relief of bladder outlet obstruction may be delayed and incomplete.

Similar considerations are appropriate if interstitial irradiation is contemplated. In the Memorial Hospital series, a significant percentage of patients required a transurethral prostatectomy and interstitial implantation of iodine 125 was delayed until at least six weeks later.[13] Since removal of large amounts of prostatic tissue precludes effective placement of iodine 125 seeds and uniform distribution of the irradiation, a transurethral prostatectomy should be limited. Often, as little as 5 gm of tissue removal may be adequate. We have performed a limited transurethral prostatectomy prior to interstitial implantation of iodine 125 seeds in 44 patients. An average of 5 gm of prostatic tissue was removed and pelvic node dissection and implantation of the radioactive seeds were performed immediately after the transurethral surgery. There have been no incidences of delayed healing of the prostatic fossa and an average of only three seeds has been lost through the urine after this procedure.

An issue that has been raised is the possibility that transurethral prostatectomy may disseminate prostatic cancer cells and promote the development of metastatic disease.[14] The fact that significant amounts of the irrigating fluid used during transurethral prostatectomy are introduced into the systemic circulation through open venous sinuses is well recognized. Whether or not viable tumor cells capable of implanting at remote sites in the body are also introduced during transurethral surgery is far less certain. Retrospective reviews have shown conflicting results. Some have suggested that patients with otherwise localized prostatic cancer who underwent transurethral prostatectomy developed metastatic disease earlier than an apparently comparable group of patients who did not undergo transurethral prostatectomy.[15] On the other hand, other series have shown no difference between groups of patients undergoing transurethral prostatectomy and those not requiring surgery.[16, 17]

A criticism of all of these studies is that, despite apparent comparability between overall prostatic size and tumor volume, patients requiring surgery for bladder outlet obstruction seem to represent a distinct group from those in whom surgery is not necessary. In the absence of good evidence that transurethral prostatectomy does disseminate prostatic cancer, most clinicians continue to perform transurethral prostatectomy when indicated in patients with carcinoma of the prostate, and it remains the most effective means for relief of bladder outlet obstruction.

Since the normal anatomical landmarks that distinguish prostatic adenoma from capsule may be lost in patients with diffuse carcinoma, the end point of transurethral prostatectomy in patients with prostatic cancer may differ from that in patients with benign prostatic hyperplasia. The prostatic fossa and bladder neck may be rigid if there is diffuse carcinomatous involvement. Often, there is less bleeding during the performance of transurethral prostatectomy in carcinomatous glands. Tumor involvement of the external urinary sphincter occurs with some locally advanced lesions and may create problems with urinary incontinence after prostatectomy. Since the anatomical plane between capsule and prostatic tissue may be poorly defined, open prostatectomy generally is contraindicated in patients with prostatic cancer.

The involution of the prostate that usually occurs after the initiation of hormonal therapy may provide symptomatic improvement in bladder outlet obstructive symptoms for some patients. The response is delayed, but most patients can expect at least some improvement in their symptoms two or three months after the initiation of hormonal therapy. Approximately 50% of patients with urinary retention will be able to void without a catheter two or three months after hormonal therapy has been initiated. Patients with metastatic disease and minimal or moderate voiding obstructive symptoms should have a transurethral prostatectomy deferred until after the results of hormonal therapy can be assessed.

URETERAL OBSTRUCTION

Obstruction of one or both ureters may occur because of subtrigonal tumor extension or bladder involvement at the ureteral orifice. Less commonly, obstruction occurs because of extrinsic involvement of pelvic nodes. Ureteral obstruction usually indicates a locally advanced tumor.

Management of ureteral obstruction depends upon clinical stage of the disease. External irradiation may provide some improvement, but response is delayed for several weeks.[18, 19] Androgen deprivation is a relatively rapid and effective method of producing tumor regression in most patients, and complete or partial relief of ureteral obstruction is usually seen.[19] The interval between orchiectomy or the initiation of estrogen therapy and relief of ureteral obstruction varies but, usually, improvement is seen within several weeks. If an LHRH analog is used, improvement in ureteral obstruction may be delayed further since castrate levels of testosterone do not occur for several weeks after initiation of therapy.

Frequently, ureteral obstruction is seen in patients who are relapsing after previous hormonal therapy. Appropriate management depends directly on the overall patient condition and expected survival. Usually, ureteral obstruction is asymptomatic although colicky flank pain may occur. If the obstruction is asymptomatic and unilateral, the best clinical decision may be to defer interventional therapy if the overall renal function is adequate. In addition, the decision to withhold interventional therapy may be appropriate for certain patients with bilateral ureteral obstruction and azotemia. In the face of diffuse, progressive metastatic disease after hormonal therapy, the duration of patient survival and quality of life after relief of ureteral obstruction may be quite limited. On the other hand, symptomatic ureteral obstruction or obstruction with azotemia should be relieved in a patient who otherwise has a reasonable quality and expected duration of survival.

Most often, relief of ureteral obstruction from hormone refractory prostatic cancer involves some sort of internal stenting. Because the obstruction is usually distal and may involve the bladder trigone, passage of internal double-J ureteral stents from the bladder is often unsuccessful. Preferably, access can be obtained through a percutaneous approach to the renal pelvis and stents can be passed in an antegrade fashion. With the advent of internal stenting, supravesical diversion by cutaneous ureterostomy or ileal conduit is rarely necessary. Similarly, ureteral reimplantation is not indicated in most patients since satisfactory renal function can be maintained by stents.

ANEMIA

Anemia is a common occurrence in patients with progressive, advanced prostatic cancer. Several factors may contribute to the profound anemia seen in some patients. Dietary inadequacy and iron deficiency may be contributory in some patients. Also, the nonspecific anemia seen in patients with chronic disease may be contributory. Of greatest significance, however, is the fact that large areas of the bone marrow may be replaced with tumor cells. The marrow of the vertebral bodies and pelvis contribute significantly to production of red blood cells, and these areas are often involved with metastatic disease.

Typically, a microcytic, hypochromic anemia is seen. Since the anemia is not of acute onset, profound anemia may be tolerated surprisingly well. However, symptomatic anemia is seen not infrequently with weakness, postural hypotension, dizziness and shortness of breath. Blood transfusions should be performed as necessary. If bone marrow replacement by tumor is an important

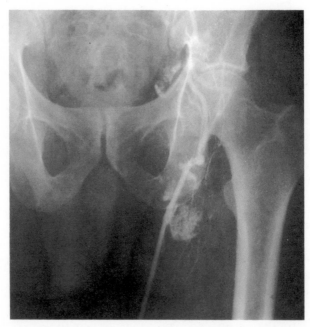

FIG 10–5.
Occlusion of left iliofemoral nervous system from extrinsic tumor compression. Flare is seen through saphenous vein only. Venous compression in deep venous thrombosis may contribute to lower-extremity edema in some patients.

factor, RBC counts may be maintained at adequate levels for only a short time and repeat transfusions are often necessary. Despite the usual advanced age, many patients tolerate hematocrit readings in the 20% to 30% range relatively well, but transfusion can be helpful in improving the overall strength and performance status of patients.

COAGULOPATHY

In addition to the anemia commonly seen in patients, other blood dyscrasias may occur in patients with prostatic cancer. A hypercoagulable state resulting in diffuse intravascular coagulation is sometimes seen with many different tumor types but is particularly associated with adenocarcinoma of the prostate. This phenomenon is usually observed in patients with progressive, terminal disease but can also be seen in those with lesser tumor burdens. The most effective treatment of cancer-associated DIC is control of the underlying disease process, i.e., the tumor. Since this frequently is not possible, treatment often is unsatisfactory and should be directed primarily at control of bleeding and correction of clotting factors.

Significant leukopenia is rarely observed in prostatic cancer patients, even in those with significant bone marrow replacement. Similarly, thrombocytopenia is observed infrequently in prostatic cancer patients. The clinical significance of any decreased platelet count can be best determined by bleeding time and, although rarely necessary, corrected by platelet transfusions.

EDEMA

Lower-extremity edema is seen commonly in patients with prostatic cancer and may occur because of tumor obstruction of either lymphatic or venous outflow. Most often, the problem can be managed satisfactorily with diuretics, compression stockings, and leg elevation. Occasionally, severe and somewhat debilitating lower-extremity and genital edema develop. In this setting, a venogram is appropriate to rule out obstruction of the pelvic veins and deep venous thrombosis (Fig 10–5). In particular, this should be considered in patients taking oral estrogens that are known to be associated with deep venous thrombosis. In hormone-refractory patients, external irradiation can be administered to large pelvic masses that compromise either venous or lymphatic outflow, although this may compound the problem rather than relieve it. A combination of pelvic lymph node dissection and pelvic irradiation often produces some degree of lower-extremity edema (Fig 10–6).

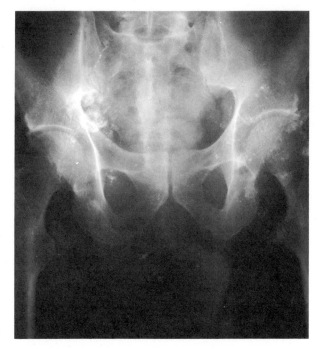

FIG 10–6.
Virtual complete obstruction of pelvic lymphatics from prostatic cancer. Extensive genital and lower-extremity edema is evident as well as retrograde filling of scrotal and penile lymphatic vessels.

SUMMARY

Many of the complications of prostatic cancer are those inherent to any chronic disease or to patients with any metastatic carcinoma. However, since therapeutic intervention favorably affecting the overall course of the disease frequently is unavailable, much of the clinical management of prostatic cancer patients involves anticipation, detection, and treatment of complications. Although a significant amount of the medical literature and attention is directed to potentially curable patients, most patients are not good candidates for curative therapy, and the most effective treatment is directed toward improving or maintaining an adequate quality of life.

REFERENCES

1. Smith JA Jr: Androgen suppression by a LHRH analog in patients with metastatic prostatic cancer. *J Urol* 1984; 131:1110–1112.
2. Geller J, Albert J, Yen SSC: Treatment of advanced cancer of prostate with megestrol acetate. *Urology* 1978; 12:537–541.
3. Benson RC Jr, Hasan SM, Jones AG, et al: External beam radiotherapy for palliation of pain from metastatic carcinoma of the prostate. *J Urol* 1982; 127:69–71.
4. Salazar OM, Ruben P, Hendricksen FR: Single-dose half-body irradiation for palliation of multiple bone metastases from solid tumors. *Cancer* 1986; 50:29–36.
5. Smith JA Jr, Eyre H, Roberts T, et al: Transsphenoidal hypophysectomy for prostatic cancer. *Cancer* 1984; 53:2385.
6. Urwin GH, Percival RC, Harris S, et al: Generalized increase in bone resorption in carcinoma of the prostate. *Br J Urol* 1985; 57:721–723.
7. Adami S, Salvagno G, Guarrera G, et al: Dichloromethylene-diphosphonate in patients with prostatic carcinoma metastatic to the skeleton. *J Urol* 1985; 134:1152–1154.
8. Foley KM: The treatment of pain in the patient with cancer. *Ca* 1986; 36:194–215.
9. Travell J: Myofascial trigger points: Clinical review, in Bonica JJ (ed): *Advances in Pain Research and Therapy.* New York, Raven Press, 1976, pp 919–926.
10. Rubin H, Lome RH, Presman D: Neurological manifestation of metastatic prostatic carcinoma. *J Urol* 1974; 111:799–802.
11. Jacovou JW: Spinal cord compression and carcinoma of the prostate. *Br J Urol* 1986; 731–735.
12. Colyer RA: Surgical stabilization of pathologic neoplastic fractures. *Curr Probl Cancer* 1986; 3:120–168.
13. Whitmore WF Jr: Interstitial radiation therapy for carcinoma of the prostate. *Prostate* 1980; 1:157–168.
14. McGowan DG: The adverse influence of prior transurethral resection on prognosis in carcinoma of the prostate treated by radiation therapy. *Int J Radiol Oncol Biol Phys* 1980; 6:1121–1126.
15. Hanks GD, Leibel S, Kramer S: The dissemination of cancer by transurethral resection of locally advanced prostate cancer. *J Urol* 1983; 129:309–311.
16. Kuban DE, El-Mahdi AM, Schellhammer PF, et al: The effect of transurethral prostatic resection on the incidence of osseous prostatic metastasis. *Cancer* 1985; 56:961–964.

17. Hoffman GS, Scardino PT, Carlton CE Jr: Effect of TURP on survival and dissemination of disease in prostatic cancer. Abstracts of the American Urological Association Meeting, Las Vegas, 1983, No. 416.

18. Megalli MR, Gursel EO, Demiraz H, et al: External radiotherapy in ureteral obstruction secondary to locally invasive prostatic cancer. *Urology* 1974; 3:562–564.

19. Michigan S, Catalona WJ: Ureteral obstruction from prostatic carcinoma: Response to endocrine and radiation therapy. *J Urol* 1977; 118:733–738.

Index